And She Lived Happily Ever After

Because every woman deserves
a happy ever after!

And She Lived Happily Ever After

Because every woman deserves
a happy ever after!

Deborah Durbin

Winchester, UK
Washington, USA

JOHN HUNT PUBLISHING

First published by O-Books, 2023
O-Books is an imprint of John Hunt Publishing Ltd., 3 East St., Alresford,
Hampshire SO24 9EE, UK
office@jhpbooks.com
www.johnhuntpublishing.com
www.o-books.com

For distributor details and how to order please visit the 'Ordering' section on our website.

ISBN: 978 1 80341 147 7
978 1 80341 148 4 (ebook)
Library of Congress Control Number: 2021951512

A CIP catalogue record for this book is available from the British Library.

Design: Stuart Davies

UK: Printed and bound by CPI Group (UK) Ltd, Croydon, CR0 4YY
Printed in North America by CPI GPS partners

Contents

Other Titles by this Author

So You Want to Be a Freelance Writer? Writing for magazines, newspapers and beyond
ISBN: 978 1 78099 492 5

Oh Great, Now I Can Hear Dead People
ASIN: B013RP7CMI

Oh Great, Now I Can See Dead People
ISBN: 978 1 78099 979 1

The Real Gypsy Guide to Fortune Telling
ISBN: 978 1 78279 452 3

Secrets to Successful Property Investment
ISBN: 978 1 78904 818 6

Acknowledgements

This book is the result of years of me observing people, questioning societal rules, and generally ranting about a lot of stuff I feel is unfair for women.

It's been one of those projects that I started a few years ago; you know the type, you think about something, get it off your chest by writing it down and get on with life; and to be honest, I never thought that anyone would be that interested in reading my ramblings. So I was over the moon when I submitted it to my publishers and my lovely editors all agreed that this was a book that *"needed to be published"*. So it is with a huge thank you to Krystina, Michael, Charlotte, and G.L. Davies, the first official readers of this book, and for believing in me and *And She Lived Happily Ever After*.

I'd also like to thank my best friend Chrissy for always being my number one fan and for supporting and encouraging me to live my best life – not to mention all the Friday nights we've had in our local, where we've often been thrown out because they want to go home.

It's with huge thanks to the other most important women in my life – my sister Hel, who will happily talk to me for hours on the phone and will drop everything if I'm having a meltdown and need a break. To my wonderful mum – you're the reason I'm here and a constant source of positive love energy in my life. And to my three beautiful, talented daughters, Bex, George and Holly-Em. You have all taught me so much about how the world is for young women today, and I hope that you continue to ask questions and refuse to put up with the Sh*t women before you have had to put up with.

Thank you to all the brave and inspiring women who have stood up and said, "Nah, I'm not having that!" It only takes one voice to create changes and enable women to live their happy ever after. I hope by writing this book every woman will realise that she has every right to be heard. She has every right to ask questions. She has every right to be seen as equal and she has every right to live happily ever after.

Introduction

What's stopping you from living happily ever after?
From an early age, girls are taught to behave and act in a particular way... Nice girls don't shout. Good girls don't demand. Being overly assertive equals arrogance. To speak our minds makes us look like troublemakers. This information is fed to us throughout our lives, and it results in women being made to feel lesser than in every area of their lives.

We're judged if we choose not to have children, we're judged if we choose to have children. We're seen as being arrogant if we're ambitious, or weak if we don't stand up for ourselves; and we listen far too much to other people's opinions of us, instead of just getting on with our lives in the way we feel will make us happy. You will never hear someone question why a man has decided to not have children, or why he wishes to remain single and live on his own, and yet women are questioned and judged every day about their views and choices.

We're judged to be weird or odd if we're not interested in having a permanent relationship with someone, or if we want to book into a hotel for a weekend of peace and quiet – again, things our male counterparts are never judged on. We're judged on what we wear, how we look, how we speak, what car we drive... aghh, the list goes on!

And She Lived Happily Ever After is an empowering and motivational guide for women that gives YOU permission to start living your life for YOU. Just because you're a woman, you don't have to adhere to the rules and patterns given to us or expected from other people. It's time to say, no, I'm not putting up with it anymore, and start living your happy ever after!

You have every right to demand happiness. You have every right to ask questions and follow a different path to the norm if you want to. You have every right to dress however you like

– hell, why not wear that tutu and feather boa when you go shopping? You have every right to live on your own. You have every right to go out with several people without labelling any of them as your significant other. If you want to quit your job and travel the world on your own, or set up a plumbing business, you can do that too, or if you want to home-school your kids, you are entitled to make that choice. YOU do not have to explain or justify yourself or your choices to anyone. Just because we've always been made to feel that we do, doesn't mean we have to.

This book draws on some of the life lessons I've learned over the years to finding my own happy ever after, which I'm passing on to you, as a reminder that you really do have the power to create your own happy ever after. They include why you need to surround yourself with radiators and not drains, how sitting back and just observing can reveal more than you know, and why the size of your audience doesn't matter, plus much more life advice I've gained over the years, so that you have the confidence to do what you want to with your life.

So, what's stopping you from living your happy ever after?

Why We Should Wait 24 Hours

We're all guilty of it – immediately reacting when something negative happens to us. It could be that a friend has said something hurtful, or your boss has asked you to work late when you've already made plans. Maybe your partner has let you down by forgetting your birthday, or the feedback you received from that interview you thought you nailed was less than complimentary. Perhaps you've told your best friend your brilliant idea for a business, and they've ripped it to pieces. Or your neighbour had taken your parking space – again. You're angry and heads are gonna roll!

But hang on a minute, my little angry one!

There's a quote that often pops up on Instagram that says: "Never promise when happy, never decide when sad and never reply when angry", and this is excellent advice to remember for every area of your life. When we are in the heat of the moment, it's very tempting to fire off an angry text or email or say something that we didn't mean – but once said, the damage is done.

If you can wait for 24 hours before you react to a situation, you will often find that whatever it was that made you so mad, doesn't really matter anymore. I'm not saying it's easy – sometimes, when we think we're right and we're feeling hurt, it takes everything in us to not react immediately. But if we react to something without looking at it from an objective point of view or the point of view of the other person, we often unintentionally make things worse for ourselves.

Let's say your best friend Alice has let you down at the last minute – again – and has messaged you 20 minutes before you're due to meet for a drink. You've had your hair and nails done, you've got your best dress and killer ankle boots on and you're already on your way to meet her. Then you receive the text telling you that your friend can't make it.

You could do one of two things: you could angrily call or text her, demanding to know why she's bailed on you again, or you could make other arrangements with another friend, or even take yourself out for the evening and contact the friend who let you down in a couple of days to check that's she's OK.

If you decide to confront her there and then when you're angry, she is going to automatically be defensive as to why she's let you down. You are going to be cross with her because you've been looking forward to this evening for ages and you feel that she's let you down again. Result? You might both say something that you'll later regret.

As disappointing as it is, if you decide to wait until you've calmed down, you will be in a better place to understand why your friend has let you down and will be more compassionate to her reasons. It's important to remember that we are all human and we all experience different emotions at different times. Your friend may be feeling anxious about going out and mixing with people, or she might have had her own awful day at work. Just because you're in the mood for going out, doesn't mean that your friend is feeling the same.

Here at And She Lived Happily Ever After HQ, I'm a great believer in the power of writing things down to get them off your chest. When you feel angry with someone and you want to scream and shout at them, grab a notebook, and write down exactly how you are feeling. You might be feeling sad, angry, and frustrated at whoever it is you're dealing with. If so, write it all down. Get it out of your head and down on paper. I actually have a notebook that a friend bought for me that says, "People I Want to Punch in the Face", specifically for this purpose.

The beauty of this is that you can say whatever it is you really feel about the other person, and they have no idea because you're not going to send it to them. Be as angry and raging as you like. Draw a really ugly picture of them, and write all the negative, angry thoughts you have about them over the picture. Feel better now?

Once you've got all your feelings written down, close the notebook and vow that you won't look at it again for 24 hours. Yes, you're still going to be pretty peeved and upset, but you won't have destroyed a relationship by reacting immediately to whatever's made you feel this way.

After 24 hours and before you decide whether to have it out with the person who has let you down or made you angry, read what you wrote down. It's amazing how often, once we've had time to calm down, we can see how ridiculous it was for us to get angry about something that happened and how little it really matters now. You may still feel justified in saying something, but you will be better prepared and calmer to deal with the situation.

In the example of the friend letting you down, you will now be much more inclined to see your friend's point of view and better able to listen to the real reason she couldn't meet up with you.

We never know what's going on in someone else's life or what problems they might be going through. If more people walked away and waited for 24 hours before reacting to a situation, the world really would be a better place. Most of what we get angry about is over silly things or miscommunication. If we just stop for a moment and wait 24 hours, it not only gives us time to calm down, but it also gives us the power to assess the situation in a more level-headed way, making us better able to handle it with more compassion and see it from the other person's point of view.

By using this skill in your everyday life, it makes you a better and calmer person, and helps toward you living your happy ever after.

It Will Pass – Honestly!

At the time of writing, we're slap-bang in the middle of a worldwide pandemic, and whilst this is new and scary for everyone concerned, it made me think about other past events that have, well, passed.

There's an old Chinese fable about a young man who rushes excitedly to his father to tell him the good news that he not only has the job of his dreams, but he has also met the woman of his dreams and is living his best life. His father looks at him and nods, then says, "It will pass, son." A year later, the son returns to his father to tell him that he's not only lost his dream job, but his dream girl has also left him. The boy's father looks at him and nods, then sagely says, "It will pass, son."

The moral of this story is that everything does pass – eventually. Whether you have lost your job, the love of your life, or you're just having a bad day, week, month, or year, it WILL pass, and things will get better for you. Honest.

I'm a great believer in learning lessons. When something doesn't work out as we had hoped it would, often when we look back, we realise that what we once wanted, wasn't that great for us. I remember in my late teens being absolutely devastated that my boyfriend at the time, who swore his undying love to me, was also swearing it to another girl at the same time. I thought my whole world had imploded. I couldn't eat without feeling sick, and I was so hurt and humiliated. But, you know what? It passed and years later, when he got in touch again, I remember feeling embarrassed that I allowed this man, who to be honest had very little going for him, to use up so much of my emotional energy. I was angry with myself for giving so much of my time to crying over him and trying to make him love me, and I felt so stupid at how I handled the situation and thinking that my life would never be the same again.

Life will always throw us curveballs. That's the beauty of life. As Dolly Parton said, "You have to put up with the rain to see the rainbow." We will be tested to the limits at times. We will fall out with friends, we will lose jobs, we will lose loved ones, we may get sick, have accidents and constant disappointments, but they will all pass. Just as the good things in our lives will pass too.

This is such an important piece of advice to remember because when things are all going well, we tend to forget that these moments are also going to pass, just as the rubbish parts of our lives will too. The philosopher, Eckhart Tolle, tells us in his book, *The Power of Now*: we only have the right here and now. The past has gone, and the future is not yet here. Yes, it can feel as though the whole world is against you when things don't go according to your plans, and it's easy to feel that life is unfair and disappointing sometimes. It's also ridiculously hard to see light at the end of the tunnel and realise that whatever you're going through right now will pass eventually and you will come out a better and stronger person, but it's worth remembering the past times when you were tested to the limits, and yet look at you now – you made it through to today.

A good exercise to do to make you realise just how quickly things move on is to write down what your life was like five years ago. You might have suffered a breakup or a divorce. You might have lost your job or had a business fail. You might have fallen out with a family member, or you might have been just going through a rough time. You might have had to move or change jobs or lost someone dear to you. Whatever negative things happened to you – and there will certainly be some in those past five years – jot them down. Now look at the list you've created. You're still here, and whilst some things might well have been traumatic and hurtful, you survived them, and you will survive whatever comes your way again – I promise.

The past year has been hard on everyone. People have

lost their jobs, relationships, mental health problems have escalated, no one has been able to get away and we all seem to be on a Groundhog Day loop, but remember, everything passes eventually, and we will all come out of this as better human beings, with more compassion and kindness to our fellow humans.

If you can try to remember that this too shall pass, you will be less affected and will be able to enjoy your life of happy ever after.

Green Doesn't Suit Anyone!

Jealousy – we've all felt it at some point in our lives. Whether it's scrolling through Insta pics of beautiful homes with their equally beautiful owners or feeling envious of a friend who always seems to get the best jobs, the best partners or just has the best life.

Whilst it is completely normal to feel a little envious of what another person has, it's very easy for this emotion to lead to spite and hatefulness of the person who has what you want. Be it a new car, a beautiful home, the latest iPhone, the perfect family etc.

It always pays to bear in mind that you have no idea what another person is experiencing, what they have been through or had to overcome in order to be living their best life, and let's be honest here, how many people post the worse parts of their lives on social media, or tell you actually their life sucks?

Everyone can manifest the life they want; I honestly believe that and it's not all mumbo-jumbo; there's a lot of science behind it (see Act As If). There's not many who are born into a life of luxury or have celebrity status, and even if they have, it doesn't necessarily mean that they are happy with their lives. They may tell you otherwise, but the thing is, being at the top, doesn't always equal happiness. It can often instil feelings of fear, vulnerability, and mistrust of other people. Just look at the number of celebrities who have sadly taken their own lives due to the pressure they've experienced of being in that industry.

How many celebrities do you hang out with at the weekend? My guess is none. Have you ever wondered why celebs tend to mingle with other celebs? It's because they often feel an inability to trust people not to tell the world about them. I personally think it must be an awful way to live if you feel that you can't trust anyone in the world to not sell a story about you.

Whilst feeling jealous is a perfectly normal human emotion and you shouldn't feel bad for any emotion you feel, I encourage you to use this emotion to better your own life, rather than try to destroy another person's reputation by saying things like, "Well, it's not like she worked for it", or "She married into money." These sort of statements, whether they are true or not, only make you look like a bitter person. It doesn't change the fact that someone has more than you, or a seemingly better life than you.

It might make you feel better about yourself for a few hours, but is it really achieving anything or benefitting your life in any way?

If you feel that pang of jealousy when a friend tells you she's got a promotion, or you see someone post a photo of the view from their balcony in Barbados, take a moment to hit pause and look at why you are feeling how you're feeling.

Psychologists will tell you that our negative emotions are usually an indication of something lacking in our own lives. When we feel jealous or envious of another person, instead of celebrating their hard work and achievements, we often feel a negative emotion because we feel inferior in some way. We feel deep down that if we had worked harder, hadn't watched so much television, or spent thousands of hours on social media, and had bothered to chase our dreams faster, we too could have what they have.

Instead of acknowledging this, it's more comfortable to direct negative feelings to another person and come up with excuses as to why they might have more than you or have a better life than you have. It takes a special person to admit that their feelings of envy or jealousy are because of their own behaviour or lack of.

And let's be honest: where does feeling green with envy get you? Yes, you can spend hours bitching about that colleague who managed to secure a six-figure contract, or your neighbour who just bought a new Tesla, but who is it hurting? Not them, that's for sure. They are just getting on with their lives, thanks very much.

Next time you feel envious of someone, acknowledge that emotion and identify why you are feeling those feelings. Secondly, instead of talking negatively about another person, how about using that energy to make your life better?

You may be feeling a pang of jealousy of your friend who is always posting photos of her exotic holidays on social media when you haven't even been able to afford a weekend away to Scunthorpe let alone sunny climes. Instead of using the energy to demonstrate your feelings of envy, use her life choices as inspiration. Make it your goal to go without your daily takeaway coffees for a year and save that money to go towards your own exotic holiday. Or promise yourself that any overtime you can get will go into a separate holiday savings account.

When your friend tells you she's just got her dream job, instead of hating on her and thinking she always comes out on top, try congratulating her and asking her if she can show you how you can follow in her footsteps. Other people are usually only too happy to help you fulfil your own dreams.

Don't waste your energy on feeling jealous and bitter about another person's success. It has no benefits and the only person these feelings are hurting is you – and green doesn't suit anyone.

What's Your World Profile?

We're all used to setting up our status and profile on social media, but what about your profile to the outside world? What's that like? How do you present yourself to others? If someone you knew had to describe you, what do you think they would say?

Here's the thing; others know nothing about us other than what we tell or show them, so how you present yourself to others is entirely up to you. Added to this, labels stick, so if you present yourself as someone who is hard to work with, this is what you are going to be labelled as. You may have just been having a bad day, but you have now shown the world a side of your personality that is probably not the real you.

Whilst it would be lovely to live in a world where we could just be ourselves, sometimes we have to adjust our personalities and our profiles in order to get the life that we want. If you're always moaning and have a negative mindset with everyone you meet, others are not going to think of you as someone who could inspire or motivate them, and they will make up excuses not to be around you. On the other hand, if you portray yourself to be someone who is positive, open, and non-judgemental, you will be surprised at how many people will warm to you and how many people will want to be around you.

I personally know a couple of people in my circle of acquaintances who life for them is one big, cynical black cloud. They find no joy in anything. If it's a sunny day, they will tell you it won't last or it's too hot. If it's raining, they will moan that the sun isn't out. It's exhausting just being in their company! And I certainly wouldn't ever divulge anything of my personal life to them. Added to this, spending time in this sort of company just makes me come away feeling rubbish and negative about everything. It's like I come away with a big, grey cloud enveloped around me. The saying misery loves company is so true!

We all have days when we feel bleurgh, but if someone were to write a profile of your personality, what would you want to read about yourself? That you're difficult or miserable to be around and to be avoided at all costs? Or would you prefer others to say you're a real ray of sunshine and that they look forward to spending time with you? I know what I would choose.

You only need to look on social media to get a good idea of what a person's personality is like. Aside from what their profile states, it's their posts and their reaction to others' posts that really tells you what they're like. If you look at someone's posts and see that they are full of arguments or they are controversial about every subject in the news, chances are you're going to think twice before you invite them into your life. And don't be thinking that you can soon convert them into little rays of sunshine – trust me, you can't. Habits are hard to break and according to neurologists, negative behaviour is a much harder habit to break than positive behaviour.

Try to be that person who is a pleasure to be with, not a pain. The more positive self we show to the world, the more opportunities we attract, and whilst we might not agree with the views of other people, if we can respect them and still be friendly, you will find that others' views of you are only good ones.

We all know that we all have times in our lives that we would rather forget or are embarrassed about, so why highlight them and bring them to others' attention? Do you really want to be that person who is considered high maintenance, difficult, argumentative, or negative all the time? The one to whom people pretend they're busy or who avoid your calls when you want to meet up?

It's all very well saying you don't care what others think,

but we all know everyone does care what others think of us and it's so much nicer to be thought of as a positive and helpful person, than someone who's a pain in the arse to deal with, and it is much easier to live your happily ever after when you show your very best profile that's not going to scare other people off. It's also much nicer for you too, and studies have shown that the more positive you are, the longer you will live. So win-win!

In order to live your happy ever after, choose to show your best profile to the world because I promise you, you will reap the rewards.

Radiators and Drains

Following on from how you present yourself to the world, I have a very good friend who is a psychologist who constantly tells me to "surround yourself with radiators, not drains" and I feel that this is good advice to carry with you throughout your life.

Radiators are those people who make you feel warm and loved. You know the ones; you can call them up at any time of the day or night and they will drop everything for you. They are the ones who are your biggest fans and who want to celebrate every little life win with you, from getting that new job to managing to get your contact lenses in without poking your eyes out.

Drains, on the other hand, are those people who literally drain you of energy. They are energy vampires and you come away feeling worse than you ever did, having been in their company for any length of time. They are the people who tell you not to get your hopes up with that new job because you'll probably hate it or point out that they knew someone who got a contact lens stuck in their eye and had to have it surgically removed – then they caught some awful disease while they were in hospital and had to have their legs chopped off.

Radiator people are kind, caring and they have your back. Even if you do make a fool of yourself, radiators will empathise and tell you a similar story that happened to them. Drains will delight in your misfortune and tell you they told you so – and by the way, did you hear about the time they switched the kettle on, and it blew up in their face?

In order to live happily ever after, it's important to look at who you surround yourself with. We often have friends who we've known for a long time, and we feel obliged to continue those relationships because, well, they've been in our lives for such a long time. But sometimes as we grow, we also outgrow people, and if these people aren't bringing anything positive to our table, then it's in our best interest to block the drain and walk away.

This doesn't necessarily mean that you have to cut off all contact with anyone who is draining your energy. All you have to do is limit the amount of time you spend with them, and make sure that when you do see them, you don't allow them to spoil your mood.

A good trick for dealing with drains is to just sit and listen to them, because drains love nothing more than talking about their misfortune and misery. If you try to defend or justify yourself with a drain, they will feed off this energy and counterattack any solution that you might have. You are not going to change their personality by pointing out how negative and draining they are. Drain people don't even have a glass half empty; they have a chipped, second-hand mug. That's just who they are, so if you do have to spend any time with them, simply listen to their moans, then walk away happy knowing that they got whatever negativity they had that day off their chest.

It's worth remembering that some people are happy being miserable and it's actually comfortable to them. If they have low expectations in life, it means they will never get disappointed or hurt.

The world will still keep moving and the drains will continue to try to pull others down the plughole with them, but while they are spending all their time doing so, the radiators of this world are happily getting on with things, living their best lives and keeping lovely and warm.

Be a radiator to others and surround yourself with other radiators!

Judging and Jumping

Like it or not, we're all guilty of judging others by the way they look and behave, and it's a perfectly natural and human thing to do. The new girl in the office who doesn't talk much could be judged as either shy or aloof. But maybe she just likes to keep herself to herself and doesn't feel the need to talk to everyone? That guy who appears to be the life and soul of every party, could be covering up the fact that he is fighting his inner demons, but doesn't feel able to tell anyone.

Just as we are all guilty of judging, we are also all judged by other people. I remember one of my best friends telling me that she hated me when we first met and said she thought I was a snob. I'm not altogether sure how she came to this assumption, or what I did to make her think this, but she did.

Don't believe the social media hype of your contacts either because that influencer who looks like she has it all, sunning herself on her sunlounger, cocktail in hand, could be suffering from validation issues due to her insecurity about herself and *really* needs people to hit that like button in order to make her feel better about herself.

I remember once interviewing a couple of influencers who ran a successful travel blog. They travelled the world, staying in all the best hotels, in some of the most amazing destinations all across the world. From their blog you would think that they had the most perfect life. The reality, they told me, was that they often had to get up in the early hours of the morning in order to catch the sunrise, and whilst they were often given free accommodation in the top hotels, it came at a price.

They had to stick to a strict photo schedule, capturing certain scenes and footage at different times of the day and night. They never got to actually experience their destination or the culture of where they were staying, and would spend hours upon hours stuck in their hotel room editing their footage. For them, although they were travelling the world, it was just a job and even though they had been to almost every country in the world, they hadn't been able to see or experience very much of it at all.

Another thing we're all guilty of, along with judging others, is jumping to conclusions. We automatically assume when a blue tick tells us that someone has read our messages, that the reason they haven't replied straight away means that they no longer like us, or we've done something to upset them. We seem to forget that other people have stuff going on too and that it could be that they had to make a phone call, rushed out to a meeting, or had just spilt coffee down themselves.

We assume that when someone is quiet and not really talking much that it has something to do with us personally, when more often than not, it doesn't mean anything other than they just don't want to talk right now, or they have other things on their mind, or they're feeling a bit under the weather. This problem is escalated by the fact that many of us only 'talk' to each other by text or messaging where there is no tone or inflection. A simple 'yes or no' in a text can be taken in so many ways because we can't see the other person or gauge how they are feeling by their tone, and no one has time to follow it with a series of emojis just to make sure the other person doesn't take offence.

So much silent information is the cause of so many assumptions in the world and we're not mind-readers! When you message someone and they don't get back to you for six hours, it could easily be that they left their phone somewhere or they've been asleep, or they've been tied up with an emergency. Don't automatically assume they are not speaking to you. And don't assume that you know something about someone when you don't.

I once had a neighbour who assumed that I was, in her words, "just a desperate housewife", when she discovered I was an investigative journalist working on a local news case. I've had a parish councillor assume I was an unmarried mother when I decided to attend my father's funeral on my own so that my husband could look after our daughter who was two at the time. I had another neighbour assume I had won the lottery when she discovered we were moving out of our social housing house and buying our own home. None of these assumptions were true, but it just goes to show you how much people jump to conclusions and assume things.

In order to live happily ever after we need to quit the judging and jumping to conclusions because none of us know what another person is doing or going through right now, and most people are so off the mark with what they think about another person.

Be Your Own Cheerleader! …

It doesn't matter who you are, or what you've done in your life, you are an awesome and worthy person, and in turn you deserve to massage your own ego. There's a line in the song, *I Know Him So Well*, from the musical *Chess* that goes: *"No-one in your life is with you constantly"* and whilst initially this could be looked at with sadness that basically, you're on your own, kid, I think it's a good reminder that we all need to be our own cheerleaders.

It is so important to celebrate all your wins, big and small, in your life, even if you just managed to brush your hair today – give yourself a high five for doing so. We spend so much time comparing ourselves to others and thinking that our lives are dull compared to some, that we forget that just staying alive each day is an achievement in itself.

When you were growing up, your parents celebrated everything about you – even if it was something as simple as using the potty for the first time, without spilling it all over the floor! Your first steps were cheered, the time you bravely stepped into the classroom for the first time, the time you finished your school exams, passed your driving test, got into college, got engaged or got your first job. All of these steps were celebrated by people who loved you and yet all the while these people are not in your life constantly – you are. Which is why it's even more important to be your own best friend and cheer yourself when you achieve something, even if it's something very simple in your life.

Too often we ignore the tiny steps we make in life to our bigger goals, such as handing in an assignment on time or getting up when the alarm goes off. If we can remember that no one in our life is with us constantly then it makes sense that we should be our biggest supporter in our life. We shouldn't have to rely on others for validation that we are a good person or deserve a place in the world. It is our right to have a beautiful life, and when we celebrate all our little wins, without having to announce it to the world, our confidence grows from the inside out.

For many women, the thought of cheering ourselves on is tainted by emotional neglect from our childhoods to the point where we simply don't know how to do it. But you have to remember that even if your parents didn't acknowledge your little wins, it doesn't mean that you should ignore them. In fact, it's necessary that you celebrate everything about you, because to ignore it is basically saying that you're not worth celebrating, and believe me, you are. You don't need validation from anyone other than yourself.

Cheer yourself on when you manage to complete that HIIT workout. Celebrate finishing work early for the week. Give yourself a high five for getting to work on time, cooking a meal by following a recipe, leaving a toxic relationship, ticking off a goal in your life, or even just managing to get a full nine hours' undisturbed sleep. No matter who you are or what you do, someone will always talk about you, question your judgement, or doubt you, which is why it is so important to be your own cheerleader.

We all come into this world with nothing, and we all go out again with nothing; it's the bit in the middle that is the important part. People will come and go in and out of our lives as we grow, so it makes sense to be our own number one fan, cheering ourselves on every single, small step of the way.

Keep it Private, People Love to Ruin Things! ...

As we've seen in the chapter about jealousy, some people have such a negative mindset that they won't think twice about making some derogatory comment about how you live your life. You could be Mother Teresa and still someone will tell you that your cross is too big!

This is why it's important to keep your life as private as possible because other people do love to ruin things for you! This could be out of jealousy, anger with themselves, or just because they're basically horrible people.

There's a similar saying, "People hate you for one of three reasons... they want to be you; they hate themselves or they see you as a threat." And there is a lot of truth to this. If someone is comfortable with their own life, they don't have the time or the energy to hate on others. They're too busy living their best life and getting on with accomplishing their own goals to be bothered by what someone else is doing. But many do.

Which is why it's important to keep what's going on in your life private from people who you know will try to ruin things for you.

We see so much of it on social media these days. The whole world is looking for validation in the form of 'likes' on what they are having for dinner or the view from their window but they forget that they're also setting themselves up to receive abuse, judgement or attack from other people. Why not just eat your dinner and look at the view in peace without the fear of people either not liking it or making a barbed comment about how privileged you are to be seeing that view, when there are starving children in Africa, or how your dinner is loaded with carbs and it's actually very unhealthy to post this sort of meal because you're just encouraging obesity?

A good friend of mine has always advised, "Live your own secret life of happiness," and I think this statement ties in nicely with keeping your life private because as we've seen people will judge you and feel it is their right to comment.

Whilst everyone is entitled to their own opinion of you, when you allow the world to know what you're doing or what your goals are, you can also be setting yourself up for others to disapprove or disagree.

You don't need validation that you are a good person from anyone other than yourself. You shouldn't care whether any of your Facebook 'friends' like the photo of the sunset you posted. To be totally free is to not care one way or the other. I understand that sometimes we like to share something that is happening in our lives, such a life milestone or an achievement with those we love, but when we're living off others' validation to make us feel happy, it becomes an addiction to living under a cloud of what other people think of us.

Some of my best times have been doing things on my own without the acknowledgement or approval of anyone else. Many times people are surprised when they find out I'm a best-selling author, or that I've travelled the world on my own, or that I built up a multimillion-pound company from nothing, because I don't feel the need to broadcast everything I do and because I fear that if I do, there will always be someone around to spoil it for me!

In order to live your happily ever after, crack on with your own life, dreams, and goals, without having to announce them to the rest of the world. You are not accountable to anyone. Not your friends, your partner or your family, and you don't need to tell anyone what you are doing if you don't feel like it. You'll not only feel happier, but you will also leave people wondering how you did it and why you didn't feel the need to tell them!

Why You Need an Alter Ego…

We all have times when the world feels overwhelming and just too much to handle, and it's at times like these when we often wish that we were someone who has more confidence or was better at these sorts of things than we were.

Enter your alter ego!

Our alter ego is someone who we all need from time to time. She's that person who when someone is rude to her, she doesn't walk meekly away apologising; she calls them out, there and then and tells them what she thinks of their rude behaviour. She's the woman who when her male colleagues shout over her, tells them that they are out of order and that her voice and opinions are just as important as theirs. She is the woman who will think nothing of expecting equal pay and equal rights, and she will fight for justice if she must.

Our alter ego is that woman who is deep inside of all of us and who oozes confidence, self-worth, and self-esteem. Basically, she's kick-ass and everything we're not. But she is there if you want her to be!

Your alter ego is someone who is the complete opposite of you and someone who you would love to be, and you can be her. All you have to do is assume her personality for you to become her.

Take a moment to write down or draw what your alter ego would be like. How different to you would she be? If you could be anyone, what different traits and personality would you have? Would you be more confident? Less forgiving? More self-assured? More of a risk taker? List all the things in your personality you feel you would love to have come to you naturally, such as the ability to speak in public without feeling anxious or nervous, or the power to command a crowd just by giving them *that* look. Perhaps you wish you were one of those people who had a witty comeback whenever someone was rude to you? Or you wish you weren't so shy when talking to people or wish you could stand up to the bullies in your life for once.

Think of the women in the world who inspire you. Perhaps you would like to have more of Helen Mirren's 'don't care what people think' attitude, or maybe you would like more braveness like Michelle Obama to publicly fight for people's human rights? Whatever you feel is lacking in your current personality, write it down.

Every time you feel a lack in confidence, or you feel anxious/nervous about something, think of how your alter ego would handle it. Give her a name and ask yourself, "What would Samantha do right now?"

Fiction authors will tell you that when they create a character, the character becomes real to them and they are often taken by surprise at how they react to certain situations, despite knowing that they, the author, has created the character and are writing their story. This is how you will soon see your alter ego. You can even find an image on Google Images of who you think looks like your alter ego and keep this in your phone for every time you need a boost of confidence.

When you assume the identity of your alter ego, you will find that you are better able to handle situations that would have previously made you nervous or anxious, and you will be amazed at how differently other people react to you when your alter ego kicks in.

We all need a little helping hand from time to time, and by adopting the traits of your no-nonsense alter ego, you will be able to handle whatever life throws at you and be living your happily ever after.

The Big M…

Whilst I've tried to make this book accessible to women of all ages to be able to identify with, there's one topic that is primarily designed for those of us over the age of 40, although I would argue that this is something that every woman regardless of age should be aware of because every woman will experience it – and that's the Menopause.

I read an article the other day that stated that women between the ages of 45 and 53 are more likely to take their own lives than any other female demographic. The links between the menopause (which most women will experience between these ages), and depression and suicide have only recently come to light, and this is thanks to some female celebrities and MPs who have been brave enough to highlight how this time in their lives has made them feel.

Just as when we begin to change from a child to a young woman, our hormones create massive changes as we enter our middle years. Aside from the physical changes, such as a lack of sex drive, weight gain, hot sweats, aches and pains, hair thinning, our mental health takes a battering to the point where many women, including myself, just don't want to be here anymore.

After a particular traumatic time in my life, I was diagnosed by my GP as having clinical depression at the age of 45. He prescribed me antidepression tablets (which to be honest just made me feel like a zombie) and suggested I get some talking therapy.

I was lucky enough to have a therapist who was a woman the same age as me, and after a few sessions of me telling her I just didn't want to live anymore and that I felt as though I would be living on autopilot for the rest of my life, she made the connection that along with the trauma I had suffered, I was also going through the perimenopause – the time when a woman's body starts changing and slowing down. My GP never connected the dots that the depression I was experiencing was associated with my age – how could he? He was male and had never experienced this.

I then began to question how many women were being diagnosed as being depressed, when in fact it was a symptom of the menopause and I discovered that depression is one of the primary symptoms. Millions of women have been told that they have clinical depression and have been prescribed medication that may not be helpful to them, and the fact that many feel that there is no way out other than to take their own lives is shocking.

Thankfully information is now filtering through, and more and more women are speaking up about how this time in their lives is really affecting them. We now have MPs such as Jess Phillips highlighting how the menopause affects women and supporting the Menopause Matters campaign, and celebrities like Davina McCall and Penny Lancaster are talking about their own experiences.

Dee Murray, founder and CEO at Menopause Experts Group, said: "Menopause affects every woman differently, but for many it can bring unpleasant physical, emotional and psychological symptoms that can be challenging to deal with. Mental health issues like depression, anxiety and stress are hard to deal with, and many women will not know that they can commonly be caused by menopause. We cannot ignore what is happening or let these women suffer.

"Women who are not aware they are going through menopause can be caught off guard by feelings of worthlessness, confusion and a complete lack of confidence. As well as those in the medical profession, psychologists, psychotherapists, and counsellors need to be trained in the basic knowledge of menopause so they can identify the root causes in patients they treat."

If you are going through a really crap time right now and you're at the age where you are experiencing menopausal symptoms, please, please hang in there. It is a horrible time for any woman; you have no idea why you feel like you do, and it just feels as though there is no one to turn to. I'm here to tell you there is and this will pass, but this is the time where you need support, so if you are feeling that life is no longer worth living, please believe that it is and seek help from other women (there are lots of good support groups on social media).

I'm pleased to hear that many schools and colleges are now making the menopause a talking point in their well-being lessons, because it affects everyone – friends, family, employers, and I hope that no woman ever feels that there is no way out in the future because of this.

If you can't find someone to listen and support you, there is a number you can text. Text 'SHOUT' to 85258 if you feel that you can't talk on the phone. This is a free messaging service with trained crisis volunteers who will text you back and help you. Please don't ever think you're alone in this because you're not.

None of us is Immortal...

I wasn't sure whether to include this topic in this book because none of us want to voluntarily think about death, but I also think it's an important topic to discuss and highlights some valuable lessons.

I watched a speech by Steve Jobs recently. It was from his commencement address at Stanford University in 2005, and in it he talks about how he dropped out of college and managed to carve his own career path to becoming known as one of the greatest technological minds the world has ever seen.

He also talked about his first cancer diagnosis and how it made him feel, and that he recognised that none of us is immortal – we're all going to die. You, me, your parents, your siblings, that bully from year nine who made your school year hell, the nice lady in the flower shop, your friends, your children, your annoying neighbour who decides to wake you up every single morning by revving his car. The taxi driver who helped you get home safely, the Amazon delivery driver, the cyclist who almost ran you over this morning... every single one of us is going to die at some point. And I don't mean to seem harsh but it's a given – we're all going to die at some point.

And the thing is, we don't know when that day might come. We know it's going to happen – although most of us put it to the back of our minds. We don't know if it will be today, tomorrow, or years in the future. We assume that we are going to have the honour of growing old, but none of us *really* know.

It always amazes me, when someone dies before they have had the chance to live to an old age, at how shocked and surprised by it people are. Saying things like, "She was taken too soon," or "He had his whole life in front of him." How do we know that? How do any of us know how long we have on this planet? We hope that we will get to our senior years, but it's impossible to know and yet we automatically assume that we're all going to continue living.

We make plans for days, weeks, months, and years into the future, truly believing that we will have the opportunity to do all the things we want to do with our lives. Unfortunately, we just don't know. Some of us will die before we get to what is considered to be the end of a normal human lifespan.

This chapter isn't written to make you go, "Oh great, thanks for that then!" It's for you to remember that none of us is immortal, and to then identify what is really important to you so that you can live your life, however long it might be, by being the happiest you can possibly be. And that means focussing on what is important and relevant to YOU.

Is it really worth your time and energy getting mad because someone took too long to move around the supermarket today? Does it really matter that your partner brought home coconut milk instead of almond? Or that your neighbour annoys the hell out of you? If we all had a label on us, telling us how long our life on earth was going to be, I bet life's little or even big annoyances would seem insignificant.

An interesting experiment I read about is to try is to calculate how many summers you have left if you were to live to the life expectancy age of 80. I've done this with friends, and we have all been shocked to realise that if we live to the average life expectancy of a human, we will only see another 27 summers! Even an 18-year-old will only have 62 summers left! It's quite an eye-opener when you look at it like that, and suddenly you begin to realise that a lot of what we get angry and frustrated about, really isn't that important anymore.

None of us can say for certain if there is anything after this life we live, or whether once we're done here, whether that is it or not. We just don't know.

In order to live your happily ever after, I urge you to work out how many summers you have left and then make a promise to yourself to try and enjoy every single moment. Don't stress if the dishes are left by the side of the dishwasher, or if your boss is the grumpiest person on the planet. These things are inconsequential compared to you being your happiest for as much time as you have on this planet. Change what you can change, do as much of what makes you happy, and surround yourself with people who are a joy to be around.

The rest is just such irrelevant stuff to give your energy to when you realise it could be you they are saying who was taken before her time.

Just Observe...

Life coach Lisa A. Romano is an expert in handling narcissists and how narcissistic people control others. Lisa advises when you're in a group setting, try to just observe other people and I think this is good advice, because you will learn so much about people when you do.

The majority of people love to talk about themselves first and foremost, and often listen only because it's good manners, and only listen in order for their turn to speak to come around.

By keeping quiet and just observing, you will learn a lot about other people, particularly in a group environment. You will learn who is assuming the role of the unelected leader – and every group has one. You will learn who the ones agreeable to that leader are, and who are the challengers in the group.

A good example of why you should just observe is when you're with someone who has very fixed opinions on a subject. These opinions can come from their upbringing or learned behaviour, and when you are dealing with someone who is adamant of their opinions, no amount of trying to get them to see another point of view is going to make any difference, so you're basically wasting your breath.

Take politics – when you meet someone who has very firm ideas about who they support in government, they will go out of their way to prove to everyone why their choice of political party is better than the opposition. You could spend hours arguing the case for the opposite party, but it really is just a waste of time. It's the same with religion. You may have vastly different views on faith; you may not even practise any particular faith, but there are people out there who will have followed a particular religion all their lives and will defend their beliefs until their dying day.

The same goes for any subject: parenting, schooling, university, jobs, careers, how partnerships should be. Everyone has a strong opinion on everyday subjects and how we should all live our lives, and we should respect that.

However, when you feel tempted to correct someone, or point out that there are flaws in the information they are spouting, you're going to be in for a frustrating time. I remember seeing an advert for a kids' drink where two young girls are playing tennis and the first girl shouts that the ball was in the lines. The second girl tells her it was out. The first girl shouts again that it was in. At this point the second girl takes a sip of her drink, shrugs, and says, "OK," and walks off the court.

The purpose of the advert was that the kids' drink gave the child the confidence to accept what her opponent was saying as *her* truth and wasn't prepared to get into an argument with her.

You can spend hours upon hours trying to prove others wrong or pointing out their flaws, but what is that going to achieve other than a feeling of superiority? They are certainly not going to thank you for pointing out that they're misinformed or wrong, and made themselves look like a complete idiot. In fact they are more likely to resent you for making them look like or feel like a fool.

To live a happily ever after, don't feel compelled to correct someone when you know they're wrong about something, or get into an argument with them. Just observe and let them get on with it. It makes for a much easier life if you do.

An added bonus to this is that when you take a back seat and just observe what's going on around you, like a fly on the wall, very few people will notice. Because they are all so busy getting their voices heard, they will miss the fact that you haven't spoken a word or revealed anything about yourself.

This means that no one really knows anything about you. You keep your anonymity, and if someone in the group were to take a quiz on you, they would be hard pushed to be able to tell anyone what you are like. And it's quite nice and rare to maintain that little bit of mystery in a world where we tell everyone everything about ourselves.

It's Their Journey, Not Yours...

Many women are natural people pleasers; we want only the best for our friends, family and loved ones and we want them to be as happy as we are and to be able to experience the best things in life too. If we're a naturally positive person, we do everything within our power to prove to those negative nellies in our lives just how wonderful life really is, and if they just listened to this podcast or read this book about the Law of Attraction, or go to this investment seminar, they too would realise that it's far better to be positive than it is to be negative... if only they would listen, damn it!

The thing is, you can't force your opinions or views on to another person, however inspiring they might be, and you were not put on the earth to fix everyone else and make *them* happy. It's up to them to decide how they want to spend their life. That is their journey, and it will be a completely different one to yours.

I know someone who, if it's a lovely sunny day, will tell you it's too hot. If the weather is chilly, it's too cold. She spends all day following people who have made their fortune and she desperately wants to work for herself, and yet she won't commit to anything, saying these people got lucky, or they are younger than her, or they had financial help etc. A constant stream of excuses as to why she can't be as successful as other people in the world.

I've tried countless times to encourage her to start her own business and I've listened numerous times to the reasons why she feels now is not the right time. I've lost count of the times I've given her money to enable her to get started in her business and each time there has been excuse after excuse as to why she can't right now.

The last time I helped her out so that she could concentrate on starting her business, I realised after a few weeks that she never was going to do it, and that maybe this is her journey and not mine.

I realised that it's actually not my job to make life easier for her and I have to live my own journey, not hers. As much as I can see her potential, no amount of me nagging her or giving her more money to get started is going to make her do it. That's her journey to travel and not mine. And maybe her incessant need to be negative about everything is her way of protecting herself from the fear of it not working out. Who am I to be the one to insist she changes her whole personality to suit me?

And it's not your journey to be other people's rescuer either. You can listen and empathise to another person, but it's not your job to rescue them or sort all their problems out. Just as we shouldn't live our lives for other people, you can't force another person to do something, no matter how much potential you can see in them. It's the old, 'can take a horse to water, but you can't make it drink it'.

Obviously you can encourage someone when they come to you with their plans to improve their life but try to draw the line at providing all the answers for them. With a wealth of information at our fingertips, everyone has the same opportunities available to them. It's not your job to persuade, cajole or solve their problems for them. That job is up to them.

In order to live your happily ever after, all that is required of you is to concentrate on you and your happiness, not assume that you have to make everyone else happy. And as frustrating as it might be, that's their journey, not yours.

Drinking Poison…

The saying goes: "Being bitter or holding a grudge is like drinking poison and expecting the other person to die." And it's worth remembering this when someone does you wrong, and you feel unable to forgive and forget.

Whether it's the idiot who cuts you up in traffic, finding out your partner has been unfaithful, discovering your best friend has taken advantage of your good nature, a family member has hurt you, or a work colleague has complained to your boss about you. To keep turning it over in your mind and think up ways in which you can get your revenge is only hurting you, not the other person.

That idiot driver isn't going to worry about their bad driving; in fact, they probably think they're a great driver. They are certainly not going to let it keep them up at night. They probably don't even remember doing it. Your ex is probably not going to think he/she made a bad choice, and will apportion blame on something you did or didn't do to make them seek pleasure elsewhere. They wouldn't have done it otherwise. That friend who took advantage of you isn't going to acknowledge that they did anything wrong and might even suggest you're actually being oversensitive about the issue. That family member who spread a rumour about you thinks they're in the right and hasn't thought to question that it might not be true, and that work colleague probably feels it's their right to complain about you.

However, by holding on to resentment and hate, the only person it is affecting is you. Unfortunately, we all have different manners and morals, and no amount of you hating on someone else is going to make them accept that they were wrong.

Albert Einstein said, "Weak people seek revenge, strong people forgive, and intelligent people ignore." I feel this is a good rule to live by. Who do you think it's hurting if you hold on to the anger and resentment for someone? You, that's who. It's not hurting the other person; they've already moved on, and once again, very rarely will someone see the situation from your point of view. We're not built that way.

Holding a grudge or hating someone can last for years and years, but what purpose does it serve to you? If you think of someone who has harmed you emotionally or physically in any way, all those feelings of hurt and anger will fester inside you. You become less trusting of letting anyone into your life because it might just happen again. But look at it this way; it's not hurting them, but it *is* still hurting you. Do you really want to give them that pleasure and power over you?

Obviously if someone has physically hurt you, you must report it to the authorities, but we're talking here about those times when someone breaks your trust or treats you badly with their words or actions.

Always ask yourself if they are really worth your anger and resentment. The problem with holding on to anger is that it's hurting you, not the other person. Do you really want to give this other person more of your time and energy when they've already upset you so much?

A good psychology tool to use in situations when someone has hurt you is to write their name on a piece of paper and pop it in the freezer. It's like you're literally freezing them out of your life, and it really works. In order to live your happy ever after, it's so much better to say, "See ya!" and get on with your own life.

Doing Your Own Thing…

We see it everywhere – in the fashion industry, in schools and colleges, in the workplace; the pressure to be just like everyone else. To wear the same sort of clothes, to secure a place at Uni, to start a relationship in our teens, to move in together, get married and have children. It's like our lives are already mapped out for us from the very beginning and it's not easy to stop and say, hang on a minute, is this what I actually want?

It takes courage and bravery to question what is considered the norm, let alone step off the predictable wheel of life. But in order to live your happy ever after, you must stop and consider if any of these practicable life things we automatically assume we are meant to do, are actually what YOU want to do.

Take for example the assumption that as a woman you will want to get married and have children. You might be one of the millions of women who actually don't have any desire to do either. I know many women who have had no intention of living with another person, let alone procreate. And it astounds me that women are asked all the time when they are going to settle down, get married and have children, and yet men are never asked this question. If men decide they wish to remain single and live on their own, that's just accepted. If a woman says she's not interested in staying in a long-term relationship or doesn't wish to live with her partner, she's questioned. Why is this? Why are men not questioned as to their marital status? Why are they not asked why they haven't settled down yet? Or when they're planning to start a family?

Unfortunately, we will never live in a world devoid of judgement, but this doesn't mean you have to make up excuses as to why you don't have children, or you don't have a 'conventional' relationship, or you choose a career in an unusual field of work, or you dress in a different way to everyone else, or decide Uni is not a good fit for you. It really isn't anyone else's business.

I remember when I decided to home-school my three children. The judgement and constant questions I got was unbelievable and I found that instead of saying, "This is a decision that we came to as a family and it's none of your bloody business," it was easier to make up excuses such as we weren't in the local catchment area to qualify for them to go to the local school or that my children had been bullied at school. None of these reasons were true, but it was easier than getting into a debate or proving to other people that what we were doing was justified. On no occasion was my husband questioned as to why his children were home-schooled.

We are so conditioned to criticism and judgement, when in reality, as long as we don't hurt anyone, what we do with our lives and how we live them, is of no concern to other people.

If you do as everyone else is doing, you will never live your happy ever after because we are all different and unique. It's quite easy to fall into the habit of taking the 'tried and tested' route in life, but you are a person in your own right. You may have similar traits to other people, but you are not them – you are you and that means you have every right to live *your* life as you want to live it.

If like Helena Bonham Carter you want to get married but live separately from your spouse, then do so. I know many married women, who since their children have left home, have made their spare room into their own bedroom. You sleep better and you don't have to put up with someone else disturbing you.

Where did this belief of sleeping in the same bed as someone else come from anyway? It's no fun for anyone, particularly if you or your partner snores, steals the duvet from you or emits a gas that smells like boiled cabbage all night long!

If you want an unconventional job, go for it. If you want to wear a sparkly tiara to the supermarket, do so. Just as if you want to return to education and become a doctor in your middle years, or you want to write a screenplay, or you want to audition for *The X Factor* or some other such talent show.

You will notice that the people who refuse to follow the norm are often the ones who are later celebrated for their unconventional lifestyles. Look at the fashion icon, Iris Apfel; 100 years old and she has always worn the most flamboyant clothes many would say were more suited to a six-year-old. Look at the shepherdess Amanda Owen – mother to nine children and works as a shepherdess on their farm. These women don't care what other people think of their 'unconventional' lifestyles. In fact, they and many other women who have chosen to live the life they want to live are now looked on as superwomen. And rightly so!

In order to live *your* happy ever after, be a superwoman and be comfortable and confident in *your* choices. Ignore any naysayers, judgers, or criticisers, because in years to come, you will be the one being admired and applauded by those who decided to follow the conventional life route.

Always Be Curious...

Albert Einstein is credited with numerous quotes, isn't he? Whether they're actually correct or not is debatable. Given the number of sayings he's been given credit for it's any wonder he had any time to discover the theory of relativity. However, one that is credited to the theoretical physicist is: "I have no special talent, other than I am passionately curious."

Being curious about the world and the people that inhabit it is a skill that few have. We tend to become creatures of habit, doing the same job, day in day out, talking to the same people, day in day out, having the same meals, day in day out.

When we are children we are naturally curious of the world that we live in. We are amazed at how things are made and how they work and how people interact with each other. As we grow into adults, this curiosity seems to leave us in favour of becoming what we think we are meant to be in the grown-up world. We stop asking questions because no one else is asking questions, and we just seem to get on with our grown-up lives of earning money to pay to keep a roof over our head.

With the amazing technology we have now, any question is literally just a click away. If you want to know what the weather is like in Vietnam right now, all you have to do is ask Google. If you want to find out how you can get a job with NASA, you can search their website.

If you have children or you've spent some time with them, you will know very well how many questions they will ask in a day! Why is the sky blue? Why is that person a different colour to me? Where do we go when we die? Why does that man have a walking stick? Why are some people blind and can't see anything? Why do flowers come in different colours?

These are just some of the questions I remember my own children asking me when they were little, of which I spent hours trying to provide the answers to.

We often assume that the way we live our lives is the only way to live life, and yet there are people all over the world, living a completely different life to the one we know. And you don't even need to travel the world to experience different foods and cultures these days. All the information is available at your fingertips. Want to know what they eat in Angola? A quick search on the Internet and you can be cooking up a dish of mufete for dinner in no time.

Added to this, we will often meet people as we go about our everyday lives who will have vastly different cultures and lifestyles to us. If we're curious and ask them questions about their lives and their lifestyles, we stand to learn that our way is not the only way to live, and we often discover new and exciting things in the process.

Be curious and devour as much information as you can, whether this be through technology, books or just talking to people. That homeless person, sitting all day with a sleeping bag wrapped around him, wasn't always homeless. He may have been someone completely different a few years ago. He would have had his own life stories to tell. The shy elderly neighbour who doesn't talk to anyone might have travelled the world and seen such amazing sights. We don't know unless we keep curious.

Added to this, being curious enhances our own lives and gives us new ideas. Perhaps you're fed up with your job but have no ideas as to what to do next? By being curious and talking to other people, you can identify your skills or learn new ones that will enable you to have a completely different lifestyle.

In Copenhagen and other countries they actually have human libraries where you can book some time with a person who has led an interesting or unusual life. The idea is that we learn more from talking to someone and listening to their life story, than we can by just reading a book. Just as you would borrow a book from the library, you book a time slot with someone and have an actual conversation with them. You might be interested in knowing what it's really like to be blind or want to know more about the challenges a transgender person lives with, or what it's really like to be a nun.

When I worked in a care home many years ago, I used to look after an elderly lady called Eve. She was what people would call 'very well turned out' – her long, grey hair tied back into a smart bun, and she was always immaculately dressed. Eve spent her remaining years in a small box room in the care home and her only luxury was to have Sky TV installed in her room.

As I got to know Eve, I discovered that in her youth she was a fashion designer for a Paris boutique. When she left France, she opened up a chain of designer fashion stores all over the country. She had lived in Kensington and hosted some of the most amazing dinner parties, with celebrities and diplomats coming from all over the world. To look at her, you would never have guessed she was a very influential and inspiring woman in her youth. To anyone looking at her now, they would just assume she was a lovely, little old lady.

In order to live your happy ever after, keep being curious. There is always something new to learn every day of your life and the things will not only open your eyes to the world, but will also make you a much more interesting person to be around.

The Size of Your Audience Doesn't Matter...

In a world of influencers and 'validation by likes' it can be hard to stand out from the crowd when you're trying to get your message to the world.

Whatever your goals are, always remember that no one was ever born an expert in any subject. Every successful person started with an idea and took baby steps to get where they are today, and each and every person is different, with different skills and that includes you.

It doesn't matter that you've started a blog and your only audience is your parents and your best friend. What matters is that you've started, and if you do something you are passionate about, your audience will eventually grow. Some of the most popular blogs and video channels with millions of readers/viewers all started with just one follower.

You may be passionate about singing, current affairs, politics, art, dogs, painting, photography, cars, macramé baskets, travelling, health and well-being, writing, knitting, cats, crosswords... whatever, but don't automatically assume that no one else is interested. In a world where there are over seven billion people, there is always going to be someone interested in what you're doing.

Take the current world interest in climate change and saving the planet. Whilst the issues have always been there, it took Greta Thunberg, just one young girl, to highlight the problems and make people take notice. She didn't initially think, I'm going to become famous for being an environmental activist. I imagine that was the last thing on her mind. She was just passionate about how humans were destroying the world, and she wanted to educate others to stop them from killing the planet.

Love or hate her, Greta is now considered to be one of the most influential thinkers in the world, known for being able to get world leaders to listen and think about what they are doing to our planet.

The Butterfly Effect or Ripple Effect is the result of a study from a number of anthropologists and scientists that states that even the smallest of actions can have an effect on a mass scale.

The idea is that when we implement a thought with an action, that action, whether positive or negative, has the ability to ripple out to a greater audience, just like when you throw a pebble into a pond. The ripples created by that action will spread throughout the entire pond.

You only have to look at subjects that go viral on the Internet to see how this works – someone posts a clip of a penguin dancing and the next minute it's like everyone in the world knows about it.

If you apply this theory to your life and what you want to do, and you keep taking baby-steps towards your goals without the intention of finding a mass audience, you will soon discover that whatever it is you're passionate about, will slowly cause a ripple effect.

You need not worry about the size of your audience right now; that will naturally follow. What is more important is that you believe in yourself, and you are passionate about what it is you are doing in your life.

The minute you let go of the need to attract an audience is when that audience will come to you. It's a bit like the Pi** off Principle (as I like to call it), which I detail later in the book – the minute you let go of needing to see a result, is the minute when the results begin to appear. In order to live your happy ever after, let go of the need for a big audience; they will come.

Detachment...

In many beliefs and philosophies around the world, detachment is when a person can successfully detach themselves from things, people, or a set of beliefs. In Buddhism they say when you are able to do this, you have found enlightenment.

Without getting into any particular religion or belief, if you can detach yourself from other people's beliefs or material things you will find it a whole lot easier to live your happy ever after.

Don't get me wrong, we all need goals in our lives, otherwise we just end up drifting along in life with no direction. However, when we attach ourselves to a particular person or an outcome, we end up becoming frustrated and discontented with our lives. If only that guy in the next office would pluck up the courage to ask you out for a drink, he would see what an amazing person you really are. If only you could earn more money to put a deposit on your own house, you wouldn't have to keep renting that flat that is riddled with damp. If only your ex could see how happy you could be together...

These are all examples of attachment. When you focus on something or someone else as the basis of your happiness, you just end up frustrated that things are not moving in the right direction for you, and ironically you end up driving those things and desires further and further away.

The book *F**k It. Be at Peace with Life, Just As It Is*, by John Parkin, shares the belief that when we stop chasing things and feeling attachment to anything, and we just allow ourselves to go with the flow and let life happen, we are better able to get the dreams and desires we want.

It's good to have goals we want to reach, but when those goals take over our present life and we feel we will be miserable until we manifest them, that's when we end up living a life of 'when x happens, then I'll be happy'.

When we detach ourselves from whatever it is we desire and accept a 'whatever, I'm happy either way' attitude, those things we want will come to us. I like to call this the Pi** off Principle – when you change your attitude to, 'I'd love such and such to happen, but if it doesn't, I'll be just fine thanks', you are not spending your life wishing. You are accepting that you will still be just fine either way.

When you hold on to attachment of anything, you create a vibe of neediness, and this is a natural repellent for any situation or person. Have goals and dreams and desires, but don't hold on to them so tightly that by not getting them it affects your life. That person you really want a relationship with, might turn out to be a right old psychopath. That college you desperately want to get in to, might not be the best one for you. That house you so desperately want, might not be your ideal home once you've moved in.

Or it might be. We just don't know. What we do know is that attaching your happiness to the outcome of something you want or feel you need takes away the happiness you could be feeling right now, regardless of your circumstances.

It's a bit like when you're waiting for a phone call or waiting for the Wi-Fi to reconnect; the longer you wait, the longer you wait. The minute you decide to detach yourself from the outcome of it and just be content with what you have right here, right now, you will find that what you want suddenly comes to you. You will find that you have a whole different attitude and vibe about you, and this is what attracts people, situations, and the things you want to you.

When I was pregnant with my first child and my landlord told me he was selling his property and had to give me two months' notice to move out, I spent weeks desperately looking for a new place to call home. I panicked as the days rolled by, thinking I must find something before the new buyers moved in and I just couldn't find anywhere that was suitable for us.

Exhausted of looking and getting nowhere, I resigned myself to the fact that if the worse came to the worst we would have to temporarily move in with my sister, despite not having a spare room to put us up, but at least it would be a roof over our heads, and that's all that mattered, so I stopped looking.

The following week a friend contacted me to say she was moving in with her boyfriend and asked if I would be interested in taking on her tenancy. Her house was perfect and in the exact location I wanted to live. The minute I detached and stopped stressing about how I was going to find my perfect home was the minute it came to me.

Fans of the esoteric could put this down to a change in energy – desperation breeds desperation and all that, but whatever your views, if you stop attaching yourself to things, you will soon see those things appear in your life. Try it and see.

F**k Validation…

From an early age we're taught about validation – if we do something good, we get validation by being told we're a good girl. If we accomplish something in our early life that is considered a good thing, we are rewarded with other people's positive approval. So it's little surprise that when we're adults we continue to seek that validation from friends, family, our boss, work colleagues, partners, even people we don't know in real life – how many times have you checked your social media to see how many 'likes' you've received for something you've posted?

The problem with validation is that the more we get of it, the more we need to make us feel OK about ourselves. It becomes an addiction. Psychologists agree that a lack of attention and validation in childhood, which comes from emotional neglect from parents/primary caregivers, results in the need for more of it in our adult lives.

Instead of living our lives as we see fit, we constantly look for approval from the outside world to make us feel better about ourselves. We post filtered selfies, our holiday destinations, our children's exam results, our new home, car, pet, promotion, all so that we can receive that fix of approval from others to assure ourselves that we are good people and are living a worthy life.

We're all guilty of it to some extent. Even if it's just calling your mother to tell her you've made a lasagne from scratch. We desperately want that 'well done!' from another person to confirm that we're a good girl.

But wait a minute. What if you didn't post that you managed to stick to your vegan diet this week? Or you didn't feel the need to tell the world how many steps you did today? Or that your boss promoted you to manager? Or that you are sipping cocktails in the Maldives right now? Would you still feel happy and excited with your life? Could you still feel content knowing that no one else knows about your achievements? Very few people when asked this question can honestly say yes, because we are so used to seeking out validation from others that we are good and worthy people.

News flash – no one really cares that you got up at 5am to do an hour of yoga, walked the dog, knitted a quilt out of llama hair, and fed the homeless all before midday. Other people are more concerned about telling others what they did that day. Granted, you could argue that by telling people all about your life events, you are inspiring others to lead a better more enriching life. I would counter-claim that the majority of people who want to shout out to the world that they were at the gym at three o'clock in the morning doing 500 squats are doing so because they want to be congratulated so that they can get their validation fix and be reminded that they are a good girl.

Whilst achieving your goals is worthy of celebration from your friends and family, in order to live your happy ever after, celebrate on your own and in your own way, because you *are* worthy in your own right. You don't need to shout it out to the rest of the world in order to feel worthy.

Another reason why it's not a good idea to seek out validation from others is that, unfortunately, there will always be someone who will want to burst your bubble and bring you crashing back down to earth with a criticism or opinion about your news, and this can destroy your self-worth in one fell swoop.

The minute you shout out about how brilliant your life is, is the minute you will find someone will say something unkind about it. This could be because they are jealous, or they think you're boasting. Of course you can limit who sees your posts or who you tell your news to, but it's worth questioning why you feel the need to tell anyone about your life in the first place. Is it because you are seeking validation and approval?

If it is, then remember that you don't need to do this. As long as you are happy with how you are living your life and you're hitting the lifegoals you want (or not, who cares?), you are more than enough, and you don't need anyone else's approval or validation that you are a good enough person.

Opinions are Just Someone Else's Beliefs...

We all have opinions on a variety of subjects – whether it's how we live our lives compared to others, or what our politics or religion are, to what books we like to read and what movies we like to watch, or how our children are brought up and everything in between, we will all have an opinion on it.

These may have been handed down to us by our parents. For example, your parents might have been life-long Labour supporters and made a good argument for why they should be in government, or we may have been influenced by our friends and family and we take these beliefs as our own without really questioning why we believe them or why they are our opinions.

Many years ago when my daughters were of school age, we decided as a family to home-educate them. This was based on the fact that the school they went to was not, in our opinion, providing them with an adequate education.

We soon discovered that many other parents didn't share our opinion. My middle daughter's friend invited her over for tea one day just so her parents could quiz her on her general knowledge in order to assess whether she was receiving a good education at home or not. In *their* opinion, they didn't believe that home-schooling could provide a child with a decent education and that was their opinion. As a side bar all three of my children got into college a year earlier than their peers. Today they all have degrees and Masters, and my eldest daughter is currently studying for her PhD.

Many people's opinions are because they know no other way of life. It's not to say that their opinions are wrong and yours are right. It's more of remembering that they are just their opinions and it's not your job to persuade another person to conform to your beliefs. Just as it's not their job to try and change your opinions or beliefs.

As a writer, I learned a long time ago that not everyone is going to agree with the words that I write and occasionally a reader will try to publicly humiliate me with a shi**y review, but that's their opinion and I respect that. I can't possibly appeal to everyone in the world and some people will just not like me and that's OK with me.

If someone doesn't agree with you, or they have an opposing view to you on something, don't try to convince them that you're right and they're wrong. It's just a waste of time and energy.

I think it's important to privately question someone else's opinion before you believe it. Opinions can often be the result of one person being loud enough to influence people around them. I remember someone writing a post about a local takeaway, saying the owner was a racist and that everyone should boycott his shop.

There was no evidence that the shop owner was racist, but the damage was done because people couldn't be bothered to question whether that person's opinion was correct or whether they were just trying to cause trouble because their chips were cold when their order was delivered. Of course we are all entitled to have our own opinions, but it doesn't mean you have to listen to them or believe them.

As long as you're not hurting anyone, own your opinions and beliefs and allow others to have theirs. In order to live your happy ever after, accept that not everyone is going to share the same opinions or beliefs as you. They are entitled to form their own views on things, just as you are. You don't need to persuade them in any way or justify your own beliefs. Allow them to believe what they like, and you do likewise.

You Don't Need to Believe the Stories...

From a young age we are told stories – not the fairy-tale kind of stories that are read to us at bedtime, but the stories that have been handed down to us from generation to generation over the years.

Growing up in a small village where, according to my parents, one side of the river lived the 'posh people' and the other side (the side we lived) were where the council house kids lived, I was always told that there was this 'them and us' divide, just as the river divided us.

It was only when I left home that I realised this just wasn't true. Neither were the stories I listened to from my teachers who told me that I wouldn't amount to anything because I walked out of most of my exams and refused to follow the 'tried and tested' formula of education.

For many women, it takes a long time before they realise that the stories they were told and believed were just not true, and that they can in fact create their own stories for themselves. YOU can be the author of the chapters in your life. And YOU don't need to believe the stories that you were told about how things should be.

If a story isn't serving you, rip it out of your book. It's only someone else's belief and that doesn't make it true for you. We all have the power to say thanks, but no thanks to what we've been led to believe from the stories we've been told.

You're not too fat to be loved just because you're not a size zero. You're not stupid because you failed your exams. You're not destined to provide for other people just because that's what your mum did all her life. You're not too old to start a business, get a degree, or become an influencer, if that's what you want to do. You don't have to have a steady boyfriend/girlfriend, just because that's what everyone else has. You don't have to live in a house if it doesn't suit you. It's your life and if you are going to live a happy ever after one, then it's wise to question what stories you've been told and whether they help you in your life.

If, for example, your father was a bit of a tyrant and your mother was treated like a doormat, it would be perfectly natural for you to attract men like your father into your own life and consequently end up feeling like your mother, because this is the story you've been led to believe – that men are entitled to treat women like sh*t.

If you come from a family of people-pleasers who never challenged or questioned authority, it's a given that you will believe that story and will become the same; avoiding confrontation with anyone who believes they are better or more powerful than you.

Any negative story you've been fed is just that – a story and you don't have to believe it anymore if it's not serving you. It's not easy to just rewrite your own story because some of the stories we believe are ingrained into us from an early age, but if they are hindering you in any way, then rip those chapters you don't like out of the book.

You might feel that even though you feel you have a lot to say, you couldn't possibly stand up on a stage and say what you want, because your mother once sold you the story that you are the shy one in the family and couldn't possibly have the confidence to do something like this. Or you were told the story that you were too loud and opinionated by your father.

The people who told us these stories were only repeating what they had heard from their parents or people around them, and they believed them enough to pass them on to us. Or they feel threatened in some way that they need to keep you on their level. That doesn't mean that you have to believe them now if they are not helping you in your life.

It feels a bit cliché to tell you that you are the author of your own story and that you are the one who can rewrite the script, but it's so true. You no longer have to believe what's been force-fed to you anymore. The people who told you that you're too shy, or you're too loud, or you were born big-built or that you are just like your father/mother/brother/aunt/uncle – anything with a negative connotation attached to it, well, you know what? You don't have to believe it anymore. If it's not serving you and all it's doing is preventing you from living your happy ever after, then now is the time to start creating your own stories and have a happy ever after ending.

Give Yourself Permission to be Happy...

I honestly feel that we should all be given lessons in guilt-free happiness from a young age.

It often seems that happiness is a payoff for something else, and for women in particular, being happy often comes at a price. Women often feel that in order for them to be happy, they have to make sure that everyone else around them is before they are allowed to be. Added to this, we often only allow ourselves to be happy if everything is going well in our lives.

As with any other emotion, happiness is just a feeling, and because we control our own feelings, we can control how we feel at any given moment. You are allowed to be happy; in fact, it's your right to feel happy right here, right now, if you want to.

Obviously, outside life events can have a huge effect on how we might be feeling at any time, but they don't have to. All the challenges that we experience throughout our lives are going to always be hard at times, but that doesn't mean that we have to be unhappy until things go right for us again.

Added to this, we often consider how other people are feeling in order for us to allow ourselves to be happy or unhappy. There will always be people you come across in life who always see the glass as half empty, or even completely empty. They are the emotional vampires who drain the joy out of everything, and this can have an effect on your own emotions if you allow it (see Radiators and Drains).

Psychological studies have shown us that emotions are addictive, and that if you are around a miserable person, you are more likely to adopt that misery behaviour in your own life. The same applies to being around happy people.

You are the one in charge of your emotions, and that means you get to decide if you want to be miserable, angry, negative or if you want to be happy, joyful, and positive. No person or outside circumstance has the power to make you anything – unless you allow it.

You could have had the crappiest day ever – your partner dumped you last night, your car didn't start this morning, your boss was an arse again and that annoying woman from HR tried her best to get your back up, but none of these people or situations are in charge of your emotions and your happiness. YOU are.

Yes, it can be exhausting when you feel as though everything that can go wrong does so, but once again, you are in charge, and you are the only one who can give yourself permission to be happy or unhappy.

If you feel that there are people in your life who are toxic and test your patience to the limit, instead of feeling angry with them, feel sorry for them. They are obviously not in control of their own emotions if they are so full of anger.

I recently had lunch with someone who on their best days is miserable and negative about everything – the country's gone to the dogs, the weather is sh*t, the dinner *I* had just paid for was one of the worse they'd eaten… you get the picture. There is nothing in life that this person ever feels joyous or happy about. You could tell them they'd won the lottery and would never have to work another day in their life, and they would tell you they're bored because they now have nothing to do. How awful to have to live like this, day in day out! People like this should be pitied because their lives are just misery and unhappiness.

Those who love nothing more than to talk about others in a negative way or try to put you down all the time? They do so because they have zero joy in their lives. But this doesn't mean that you have to allow them to take away your joy and happiness.

In order to live your happy ever after, just observe these emotional vampires, say nothing, and feel sorry for them because they will never have the experience of happiness and that's really kinda sad when you think about it. And in the meantime, give yourself permission to be happy, because being sad and miserable all the time brings nothing to the table for you.

Assume a New Identity…

Unfortunately, it's as old as time itself: if you're a woman, dealing with men or with something that is predominately male dominated, there is a good chance that you are going to get ripped off, simply for the fact that you are a woman.

Any woman who drives will have a story of taking their car to the garage and being blinded with mechanical mansplaining jargon about what 'needs' doing to their vehicle, and we know they would never speak to a man like this. I've worked in property development for many years and the number of times I've been overcharged for work by greedy contractors who assume that they can get away with charging double because I'm a woman and I probably won't question it, because, well, what do I know?

It's frustrating and downright wrong, but there is a solution to getting the same treatment as you would if you were a man and that's to assume a new identity for such incidents.

As I write this, I feel as though I should duck because I know many of you reading this will be screaming, "Why the hell should we do that?! We have every right to be treated the same way as our male counterparts!" And I agree, we do have every right, but welcome to the real world!

It doesn't matter how many times we wave the equal rights flag, we are unfortunately still in a culture where women are treated very differently to how a man would be treated in the exact same scenario. It's a fact, I'm afraid. If you don't believe me, try it out for yourself. Ring a garage about a fictional problem with your car or call a builder with a query about a dripping tap. Then ask a man to do the same and see how your experiences differ.

I personally know of one businesswoman who got so fed up with not being taken seriously by men that she set up a fake male email address. She said the responses to her 'male identity' emails were markedly different to those when she had emailed from her own email account.

I recently had to have some electrical work carried out on a property I owned. The male electrician I emailed quoted me a staggering amount for it, saying he would have to channel the cables into the walls, replaster them and paint them. I've renovated properties for over eight years, so I know that it's possible and cheaper to trunk the cables, instead of channelling them into the walls. I decided to email this chap again but from my company email which is just an admin email address and I signed it as "Paul – Head of Property Management". 'Paul' asked why the electrician couldn't trunk the cables in the property and requested a new quote... which arrived within minutes and was a third of what he had originally quoted me.

If you're going to get the same treatment as a man, *sometimes* you need to assume the role of a man in the same position as you. This isn't as hard as you think. In the age of the digital world most people communicate via email or message, so you don't need to adopt a lower voice or grow a beard!

Set up a separate email address as 'Mark.admin@outlook.com' or something similar if you are running a business, and use this address whenever you need to correspond with someone you've had trouble dealing with in the past. You will be amazed at how different your request or complaint is treated. Funny enough, not only will your query get answered quickly, but you also won't end up getting ripped off or fobbed off due to your gender.

It's also important to remember to write your emails as though you were male. Women and men correspond very differently, so pay attention to how you write any messages. Men are very direct in their texts or messages and don't tend to end with 'lots of love' or 'xxx', so bear this in mind when you're writing a message in your new male identity.

I agree that this shouldn't happen in this day and age, but it still does, on a daily basis and we shouldn't have to assume a male role in order to get the same service, but in order to live your happy ever after, sometimes you just have to play the game and give yourself the advantage in life.

I would love to say just be who you are in these sorts of situations, but unfortunately women are still not equal to men in so many ways, and no amount of flying the feminist flag is going to change this. You see it day in, day out from politics to the workplace and most definitely with general day-to-day things.

So, if you're in a situation where you feel you are being ignored or you feel as if you are being overcharged for something because you're a woman, try adopting a new male identity.

When You Treat Someone Like a Celebrity, They Will Treat You Like a Fan…

I'm all for admiring people who have achieved what they want in life and celebrating their achievements and success, but you have to be careful when you treat someone like a celebrity… because they will always treat you like a fan.

For example, you may have met the perfect partner. Everything about them is magical and you can't think of any faults, and even if you can, they are such adorable faults that you can't really call them faults; they're just quirky foibles. You get the picture.

The problem with this is that the more you put someone on a pedestal, the more they will eventually end up looking down on you. You will have bigged them up so much, that they have no choice but to believe that they are better than you. Any relationship you have, whether it be romantic or otherwise, should always be equal. When one person in that relationship feels that the other person is above them in some way, that relationship will always be unbalanced.

There's another saying that says you should never meet your idol, because you will end up getting disappointed by what you see. It's important to remember that we are all human beings, and we all have positive and negative traits. It doesn't matter whether you're the roadie or the pop star, we all have the same problems, insecurities, confidence issues, and the same basic human needs.

My grandmother often said, "Everyone has to wipe their own bum," which was her way of saying that no one is any better than you and you should never put yourself in the position of allowing yourself to treat someone else like they are above you. If you do, you will always be considered lesser than them in yours and their eyes.

Narcissists are a prime example of being able to manipulate others into believing they are above you. They charm their way into your life, and before you know it, you are in adoration of them and you have become their fan, whilst they claim celebrity status in your life, eventually adopting the role of puppeteer as you become their puppet.

When we make someone a celebrity in our lives, it diminishes our own personality. We believe a person to be so elite that we can forget that we are just as equal and just as special as any other person in the world. And oftentimes, when we've given another person a celebrity status, we can find ourselves very disappointed when we eventually realise that they are just regular human beings, just like us.

To live your happy ever after, you need to realise that YOU are the celebrity in your life. You are a unique individual who is worthy of celebration for everything you do in your life. You shouldn't need to put anyone on a pedestal other than yourself.

I think it's important to remember that those people who you regard as being successful in life, whether it's your boss, a work colleague, a friend, a partner or even an award-winning actor or pop star, they all started off just as you did – as a tiny human being. They didn't have any particular special superpowers when they were born. They just decided on a certain direction to go in life, and they went for it. Just because they might now be successful with adoring fans, it doesn't mean they are any better than you are.

But the minute you treat them like a celebrity, is the minute you will be treated like a fan.

Don't Justify Yourself…

In order to live your happy ever after you do not need to feel as though you have to justify yourself – ever! Whether it's your decision to buy a new pair of shoes or hand in your notice at work, you do not have to justify it to anyone, and if you feel as though you do, then I'm here to ask you, why?

For far too long, women have felt that they always have to justify their choices and their decisions – you don't. There is no rule book or law saying that you have to justify anything that you do. So long as you don't go around intentionally being unkind to other people, because let's face it, that's just shi**y behaviour, whatever you want to do, do it. You don't have to explain your actions or your reasons for doing anything.

It always amazes me how much energy people give to other people instead of giving the same amount of energy and attention to themselves. If we make a decision about something in our lives we feel as though we have to justify it with a reason or an excuse. We don't seem to be able to just decide on something and be done with it. We feel we have to explain our thinking behind it.

Example: it's Friday night and as with Friday night for the past 10 years, it's the night that you get together with some friends at your local pub for food and drinks and a catch up of the past week's events in your lives. This Friday you don't feel like showering, getting dressed and putting on your best-happy-face. All you want to do is change into your joggers, eat a huge amount of carbs, and lie on the sofa watching the telly.

But instead of sending a message to your Friday Night WhatsApp Group, you sit there thinking of all the plausible excuses as to how you can justify cancelling… Say you have to work late? No, Becky from up the road saw you return home early this evening. Tell them your cat is sick and needs to go to the vets? No, that might tempt fate, and besides, Molly is good friends with your cat's vet. Dodgy tummy from food poisoning? Yep, that would work well. No one wants to be with someone with a dodgy tummy, right?

Why do we feel we have to justify ourselves? Why can we not just send a message saying, "Sorry, not going to make it tonight, have fun!"?

The reason we feel we have to explain or justify our decisions usually comes down to us not wanting to be thought of in a bad light, so we feel the need to explain away our actions. When we attach an explanation to a decision, other people think, "Ah, right, that's why she doesn't want to work there anymore! Makes sense." Or whatever the decision might be.

A justification makes sense to people and makes it all alright between all concerned. There is usually a reason why we make life decisions, but that doesn't mean that you feel that you should justify those reasons to others. It's no one else's business if you want to start a completely new career, leave your partner, or not want to go to Friday Fun Night. **You do not have to justify your decisions or your life to anyone and it is no one else's business anyway!**

In order to live your happy ever after, try not justifying yourself to anyone. If you don't feel like going out, just say you don't feel like it. If you want to hand in your notice, just do it with no justification attached. Yes, it will confuse people, but hey, that's a them problem, not a you problem.

And if you find you have difficulty in stopping yourself from justifying everything and need to ease yourself into it, read the next chapter on ideal excuses to use when you don't want to do something, but can't just say no, without justifying it.

Can I Get Back to You on That?

I realise it's hard to suddenly implement the need to justify yourself and not everyone can do it without feeling an overpowering need to explain themselves, so this chapter is a helping hand to ease you into the process of not justifying yourself.

Because we don't want to offend other people, we will come up with all manner of excuses and reasons as to why we don't want to do something another person wants us to do. The problem with this is that we can end up living a life of constant people pleasing and this will just lead to resentment if you continue to do this.

There is an easier way to begin claiming back your power and living your happy ever after: by slowly introducing saying thanks, but no thanks to other people's requests. If you feel that you don't yet have it in you to stop justifying yourself, try the following...

- **Can I get back to you on that?** This works for any request from another person, whether it's your boss asking if you're available to do overtime, a friend asking if you can water her plants while she's away on holiday, or someone asking you out on a date. You're not saying no, you're just asking for time to think about it. Oftentimes just by saying, "Can I get back to you?", the other person will go and find someone else to ask, and if you don't want to do whatever it is that's being asked of you, you get back to them and say you're sorry, you checked and you can't do it. You don't explain why, you just can't.

- **I'll check my diary.** Again, this is another stalling tactic that works well and gives you a bit of thinking time to work out whether you want to go on that camping weekend that you know you're going to hate. By saying you need to check your diary, you are effectively saying, no, that doesn't work for me, but other people will psychologically assume that you are so super busy that they will appreciate you taking the time to check if you can make time for them. And if you really don't want to go, you simply say you're sorry, but you have something else booked in on that day/weekend/month/year.

- **I'd love to, but I can't.** Again, you're not directly saying no to a request, nor are you justifying the reason to another person's request. In fact you are saying that you would have loved to man the raffle for the village fair, but there is a reason why you can't. You don't need to explain that the reason is that you have better things to do with your weekend off, you've said no, with no justification on your part.

- **Can we talk about it later?** Whilst at first this might sound as though you're just avoiding the subject, it's actually a good way of deflecting a request from yourself. It will also make the other person think as to whether they can get what they want from you. The more urgent their request is, the more likely they will find someone else who is available immediately and will have forgotten they even asked you.

- **Maybe.** By saying maybe to a request you are a) not saying no, and b) not justifying a reason why you are saying no. You're saying maybe yes, or maybe no. Again this gives you the thinking time you need to consider whether or not you want to oblige. It also makes the other person feel good that you haven't said no outright; that you're thinking about it. After saying maybe and leaving it for a while, you can then use the I would have loved to, but I can't... saying.

- **Change the subject.** This is a classic psychological trick to avoid answering a question or avoiding having to justify or explain yourself. You simply change the subject, and it works every time. If someone requests something from you and you don't want to do it, just change the subject to something else. The key here is not to point at something over their shoulder and shout, "Look, there's a bear!" Rather tell them some gossip or a fact that will shock them. The fact that you have changed the subject will throw the requester off and they will feel as though they can't ask again.

- **Sorry?** When someone asks something of you and you don't want to say no, but you also don't want to feel that you have to justify why you don't want to do it, simply asking them to repeat the request will make them rethink what they are asking of you. For example, your friend has again asked if you can lend her some money until she gets paid at the end of the month. She asks you every month and you've always obliged. When she asks again, just say, "Sorry?" and raise your eyebrows as if you are incredulous that she would ask you again. Nine times out of ten they will try to justify their request and feel very uncomfortable about asking you again.

Two additional psychological tips to remember when you are dealing with difficult people who won't take no for an answer. One is to look at their forehead, rather than their eyes, when you're talking back to them. This makes people feel extremely uncomfortable and self-conscious because we are so used to direct eye contact.

If someone is giving you grief and won't let things drop, throw them off guard by telling them they have something in their teeth or around their mouth. Again, this will make them feel silly and self-conscious, and they will quicky change the subject – once they've checked themselves in the mirror!

Forgive, But Don't Forget

Unfortunately, unless you live a very sheltered life and have no interaction with other people, you are going to get hurt at some point in your life. It might be in a relationship. It might be the words that someone says to you. You could, like me, fall victim to a rogue builder, costing you thousands of pounds, or it could be an online scam, or you could be trolled for something you've posted on social media, or someone you trusted steals from you.

Unfortunately, this is life. Not everyone is going to be as lovely and as kind as you are, and there are some people out there for whom greed gets the better of them, and there are some who are just plain horrible, selfish people.

When someone disappoints you or lets you down like this, it's hard not to wish ill feelings on them and go and look on Amazon for a cauldron so that you can hex the hell out of them, but hold on there for a moment, my little witchy one!

As much as it's perfectly natural to want to hurt someone who has hurt you, there are a few reasons why it's not a good idea. For one, you could land yourself in trouble and end up being the one having to explain to the police as to why you slashed all the tyres on your ex's car. Secondly, and more importantly, holding on to that anger is not hurting the other person. They are not going to feel the remotest bit of shame for hurting you. They've done what they've done and have moved on. As with the chapter on drinking poison and expecting the other person to die from it, it just isn't going to happen.

Added to this, I'm a firm believer in karma, and eventually that person who hurt you will get justice in another form. The builder I mentioned who stole thousands of pounds from me eventually went bankrupt and had everything taken from him, including his house. Also, we should really be feeling sorry for these types of people because eventually they run out of people to hurt and end up living very lonely lives.

For your own well-being it's important to learn how to forgive someone who has hurt you. If it really is bothering you to the extent that you can't function without thinking about them, then find a confidant you can trust and get it all off your chest. No amount of reliving it is going to make a change to what happened, and even if the person apologises, it's not going to make any difference, so I beg you to forgive them because when you do, you have your power back. They no longer have a place in your mind because you have forgiven them.

The most important thing to remember once you have forgiven the hurt you've suffered is to not completely forget it, because if you do, you could easily end up on rinse and repeat, and you will suffer all over again with someone else hurting you.

When we learn to forgive, but don't forget, it means that we are aware of not repeating what happened. We learn to not allow people to walk all over us, not to lend money to friends, or make sure we check out every tradesperson as if we were a private investigator. We remember how we were cheated on before and we don't allow it to happen again. This is the art of forgiving but not forgetting, and will help you to live your happy ever after.

It's also equally important to not allow a bad experience like this to ruin you and make you feel as though no one can be trusted. When I suffered at the hands of the cowboy builder, I was furious, and it made me feel as though I couldn't ever trust anyone again. My lovely lawyer reminded me "never stop being a good person because of bad people" and I think this is good advice, but still don't forget entirely.

Succeed in Silence

We looked earlier at how important it is to keep things to yourself and this is another reminder that if you are wanting to succeed in something, then do so in silence.

We all have goals that we'd like to see come to fruition before we die, and studies have shown that when we tell everyone about those goals, we actually hinder them.

The problem with telling people what you hope to achieve is that not everyone is going to be a fan, particularly if your goal is something that is out of their comfort zone or might actually affect them in some way, and we subconsciously take on other people's views, which can then prevent us from attaining them. Doubts begin to set in, and you start to question yourself and whether you're capable of achieving your goals all because you've mentioned it to someone else and they've been less than supportive, or they have laughed at your ideas or told you that it's an impossible dream.

For example, perhaps it's been a lifelong dream of yours to get your pilot license and fly around the world, and you tell your sister – who just happens to be terrified of flying. Because of her narrative of flying, she's probably not going to be 100% supportive of your decision and may even make you change your mind by pointing out how difficult it is to become a pilot or how much it's going to cost you in time and money.

Another reason why you should succeed in silence is because the minute you tell someone else about your plans, you put pressure on yourself to complete the task. Perhaps your goal is to join a gym and get fit again. You tell everyone that this year is the year when you will lose that stone you put on during lockdown, and you sign up, take your introductory class and then... well for some reason, you stop going. It's too cold to go out, you don't feel like working out, and before you know it, the weeks have flown by, and you realise you haven't been to the gym once. And that's perfectly OK, but now other people are going to keep asking if you're still going to the gym! If only you'd kept quiet, you wouldn't have to feel the need to explain why you haven't been back to the gym – although as we know, you don't actually have to justify anything to anyone, but still there's that feeling of, "I wish I hadn't said anything in the first place."

Added to this, there are some people who will want to wee on your bonfire if your goal is something that they have always wanted to achieve themselves. Jealousy will often rear its ugly head in some people and they will give you their opinion on how you should live your life if you let them.

There's something quite exciting about keeping your plans to yourself. I have a friend, who at the age of 50, started learning to drive in secret. She had always relied on her husband for lifts and one day a friend of hers said she should have a go at driving. It would make her more independent, and she wouldn't have to rely on her husband if she wanted to go out anywhere.

My friend used to walk to the end of her road to get picked up by her driving instructor, telling her family she was popping out to see a neighbour. Instead she would have an hour's driving lesson.

Her family couldn't believe it when she came home one day with her driving license in her hand. Had she told them beforehand, they would have told her not to bother because her husband would take her anywhere she wanted to go.

It's a great feeling when you accomplish a goal in silence, and you can then show others the results. You might want to change jobs, start a business, move out of the area you live, write a novel, move to Nepal and become a sheep herder, learn a new language, or start a degree. Whatever your goals are, keep them to yourself until you reach them and succeed in silence.

Defriending

Very few of us still have friends from infant school or even college and Uni, and there's a reason for this: we grow up and we grow out of people. Often the only reason we befriend someone is because they are in the same class as us or we share the same house. Sometimes we form close bonds with people we work with, but when they get another job, the relationships fizzle out – but that's a good thing. If we only ever stayed in touch with our friends from childhood and ostracised everyone else, we would not have the opportunity to meet new and interesting people.

When I worked in an office, Jen, a lady who was retiring after 25 years of working there, was thrown a retirement party. When she was presented with her gifts and flowers from the rest of the staff, she got up and made a speech.

"I know many of you have come up to me over the past few weeks, with invitations and promises of us all keeping in touch after I leave here, but let's be honest and not pretend, shall we? We all know that the only thing we have in common is this office and we all know that despite the promises of getting together every month, it just isn't going to happen. I wish you all well, but I probably will never see any of you again and I'm fine with that."

Many from the office were upset by Jen's speech, but she was exactly right; the only reason we were all friends was because we had something in common, which was that we all worked in the same office. Outside of that, we all had our own lives and friends of our own. She wasn't being mean she was just being honest, and she was right because I've never seen or heard from Jen again.

Just as you probably don't have anything to do with your childhood sweetheart, it's healthy to move on from friends who you've outgrown and that goes for them too. Unless you're very lucky you will find that the friends you had years ago, you have nothing in common with anymore. We all go in different directions as we grow up and that's how life is meant to be. We're not meant to stick to seeing a select few people just because they've been in our lives for a few years.

Another reason to defriend people is when you realise that you spend more of your time disagreeing with them than you do agreeing with them. Our upbringing and influences will result in our views of the world as we see it and they may differ to another person you know. If you suddenly realise that you have less and less in common with a friend, then maybe it's time to defriend them? If they're not supporting you and just causing you misery or anxiety or you find that you have become their emotional punchbag, then in order to live your happy ever after, you need to wish them luck and say cheerio.

Signs that you need to defriend someone are when they no longer want you to feel good about yourself. Even when they give you a compliment, it has to have a little negative attached to it. Or when someone doesn't want you to feel good about yourself and tries to undermine you. They feel the need to belittle, drag-down and humiliate you in order to make themselves feel better and reinstate the hierarchy in the relationship. These 'friends' are not really your friends and you don't need them in your life.

When you feel you need to defriend someone in your life, you don't need to announce it to them and throw a divorce party. You don't need to do or say anything. The other party will likely be feeling the same, and if they don't and they keep asking to meet up, just tell them you'll get back to them. As with a relationship, if it's not making you grow together, then you are better off putting it in the past so that you can both grow and flourish.

Once a year it's a good idea to go through your friend groups and check whether or not they are bringing anything to your table anymore. Just because you joined that Bumps & Babies parent group when you had a toddler, who is now a fully-fledged adult, doesn't mean you have to keep in touch with all the other members if you're no longer getting any enjoyment out of seeing them.

Just as we discussed in the chapter about Radiators and Drains, if seeing someone feels like a chore, rather than a pleasure, it's time to delete them from your phone and make room for new people to come into your life.

True Colours

Sometimes we think we know someone and then they do something that makes us realise we don't really know them at all – and it sucks. Narcissists and manipulators are classic examples of this, but it's not just those who have narcissistic tendencies; many people will show you their true colours when they feel threatened, or things don't go their way in life.

Take for example your best friend – you've been through everything together. You've celebrated and commiserated with each other since your childhood days and you both vowed nothing would ever come between you. Then one day your best friend asks you out for a drink. You tell your friend you can't make it that day, so you suggest your best friend asks another friend you both know.

Later in the week, the other friend lets it slip that your best friend didn't believe that you were busy and spent the evening running you down. Now, we're all prone to a bitch sometimes, but this is your best friend! You and her against the world, right?

Instead of accepting that you declined her invitation and enjoying her evening out without you, she showed her true colours and bitched about you to the other person. And unfortunately it happens in life. No matter how much you love someone, when they are faced with the choice of sticking by you or saving their own arse, invariably they will save their own, rather than save yours.

A friend of mine once employed her best friend's husband to build a new conservatory for her. He was out of work, and she thought it would help him. He said he would do everything from designing it to supplying the materials. She told him he had to stick to a budget, but as the weeks went on, she seemed to be having to add more to the budget because he said the supplier's prices had increased since his original quote.

After giving him another £3000 on top of her original budget, she asked him next time he came to work if he could bring all the receipts with him. And this is when it got nasty. He wanted to know why she wanted the receipts. Did she not trust him? He got really angry about it. He kept putting off letting her see the receipts from the suppliers and left the job half finished. He showed his true colours when he felt he was going to be found out for taking more money from her. This then spilled over to her friendship with his wife, who was understandably torn between standing by her man or her friend.

In psychology they term this behaviour as fight or flight. When someone is confronted by another person, that person will either fight (get defensive, aggressive, and angry) or they will want to get away from the situation as quickly as they possibly can. And this is when they will show their true colours.

This was more prevalent when I worked as an investigative journalist. The minute I had to ask difficult questions, the other person would either get defensive or angry with me. They would show their true colours, which would be completely different to how they initially portrayed themselves.

Obviously, it would be very sad if you had to be suspicious of everyone you met in life, but in order to live your happy ever after, always bear in mind that even the people you trust most in your life will often show their true colours when faced with a something that might threaten them in some way.

Act As If

Everyone from Plato to Oprah has the belief that when we act as though we already have something or act as though we are living the life we wish to live, we manifest that into our reality. We also do this for the things we don't want. Whatever we give our attention to, we create it for real in our lives.

We think that we won't have enough money until payday and guess what? Suddenly our car breaks down, or an unexpected bill pops through the letterbox and we say, I knew that was going to happen! Yup, because that's exactly what you believed would happen and what we believe manifests itself. It's a pretty powerful thing, and also a guaranteed one.

So imagine if you turned it on its head and acted as though you had everything you ever wanted? Given the metaphysical theory that our thoughts become things, how do you think your life could be? If you can create unexpected bills, you can create unexpected income, or your dream job, or owning that 19-bedroom villa in the South of France.

It's called 'acting as if' and you might be surprised to know that when you act as if, your brain doesn't know the difference between something being an act or being real, unless you tell it so.

For example, if you want to be a millionaire and you begin to act as if you are worth millions and living a millionaire lifestyle – taking yourself out to The Ivy and acting as if it's a place you frequent all the time (even if you only have a drink there), test driving a brand new Tesla and acting as though you are rich enough to buy one – your brain can't distinguish that you are not that person, unless you tell it otherwise.

Want to be a best-selling novelist, living in a loft apartment in New York? Then use your imagination and act like you already do. You will suddenly find that you attract opportunities that will lead you to that very lifestyle.

You might suddenly be offered a voluntary redundancy package which would mean you could rent a place in New York and have enough money to not to have to get a job for a year, giving you plenty of time to write that best-selling novel. Want to become a life coach and work from home? Then act as though you already are – clear out the spare room for your consultation room, follow other life coaches online, study a course (many are free online), mention that you are training to be a life coach to friends/colleagues. Before you know it, you will be that life coach with a diary full of appointments.

People tend to think that acting as if you are living your dream life is enough to get that dream life, and this is where most people fail and end up disappointed. Acting 'as if' is the first step, but the minute you do, you will notice that opportunities come your way as if by coincidence. It's then up to you to act on these.

By way of an experiment, think of a particular car you've always wanted. Imagine the colour, the trim and everything about that car. Alternatively, think of a vehicle that you don't often see on the roads, like a bright pink lorry. I'll bet you anything, the minute you think of it, you will start to see the vehicle you pictured in your mind. It works every time. When I was thinking of buying a red Mini as my next car, that's all I saw – red Minis everywhere; in the supermarket car park, passing by my house and even parked up at the bottom of the Snowdon Mountains!

It's great fun to play this game, like thinking of the most outlandish vehicle such as a lime-green campervan – and trust me you will see one. This just goes to show the power of our mind is to be able to manifest something. The fact is that that lime-green campervan was always going to be there. You didn't just magic it up by thinking about it; rather you have trained your mind to notice and look out for it, and this applies to anything in your life. What you focus on you bring into your reality.

Once you've proved to yourself that this system works, you can start to work out what it is that you want in your life. Write down how you want to be living your life (see the Perfect Day chapter). Be careful to not write down what it is you don't want, because this will just give you more of what you don't want! For example, if you say you *don't* want to be financially struggling every month, you will just attract more of *not* wanting to struggle financially. Rather, write down that you are now financially independent and that all your money needs are met.

If you are fed up with being single. Don't say you wish you could meet the man/woman of your dreams, because you will always be wishing that you could meet the man/woman of your dreams. Instead write down what your perfect partner is like. What are his/her personality traits? What do they look like? How do they treat you?

You really can manifest anything and everything you want when you act as if you already have it, and you open up so many new possibilities and opportunities for yourself. It's your right to live happy ever after, so claim it!

Don't Fix

It's very tempting to try and fix people and make their lives happier and easier for them, but this is something that it's best to try to avoid doing, especially if like me you're a people person and can see the potential in everyone.

The thing with trying to fix everyone and make them happier is that it can often backfire, and you can end up feeling resentful and angry. There's a famous fable that goes...

Once upon a time, a young girl was playing in her grandmother's garden when she noticed some butterfly cocoons getting ready to open. She watched the first butterfly trying to come out of its home. It struggled and took a long time. By the time the butterfly got out, it was exhausted. It had to lay on the tree branch and rest awhile before it could take flight. The little girl felt so terrible for the little butterfly, who had to go through so much of a struggle just to get out of his little cocoon.

When the little girl saw the second cocoon getting ready to hatch, she didn't want it to go through what the first butterfly did. So she helped open the cocoon herself and took the butterfly out. She lay him on the branch and saved him from the struggle. But the second little butterfly died, while the first little butterfly who had fought so hard took off into the sky.

Distraught, the little girl ran to her grandmother, crying. "What happened? Why did the second butterfly die?" she asked.

Her grandmother explained that butterflies have a liquid in the core of their body, and as they struggle to get out of the cocoon that liquid is pushed into the veins in the butterfly wings where it hardens and makes the wings strong. If the butterfly doesn't push and pull and fight to get out of the cocoon, his wings won't be strong enough to fly, and the butterfly dies.

"Without the struggle, there are no wings," Grandmother said. "Just like it will be with you, child. In life you will go through hard times. But it is the hard stuff, the struggle, that will help you grow, and help you learn to fly."

"But won't it hurt?" asked the little girl.

"Sometimes, things will hurt. Sometimes, things will be hard. But one day, it'll all be worth it. And you'll learn from all your struggles – they'll teach you how to fly!"

Struggles make us stronger, they teach us, they empower us, they connect us.

And it is an individual's journey to travel, not your responsibility to make it easier for another person.

By all means make suggestions when someone is down on their luck. Maybe a friend has lost her job and is worrying how she's going to pay her rent. It's not your call to pay it for her. In my experience when you do this, you will continue to do it over and over again and she will not be learning the importance of standing on her own two feet if you are constantly bailing her out. And often when you help someone out financially you later discover that they used the money for something else entirely. Not to mention doing this completely changes the dynamics of your relationship with them.

If you've ever been to see a therapist, counsellor, or life coach, you will notice that they don't try to fix you. It is always up to you to try and find the answers yourself. As with the struggling butterfly, other people need to have the chance to figure things out for themselves. You can be an inspiration to them by fixing yourself and demonstrating that anyone can fix themselves, but in order to live your happy ever after, try not to rush in and fix everyone because we all need to experience the rough times if we're to grow and flourish.

You Do You

This is one of my favourite sayings that my daughter uses all the time and is basically saying that you accept someone else's life choices, even if you don't agree with them, and I think it's a good rule to live by if you want to live happy ever after.

As humans, we can often have very similar traits – for example, whatever your age, you will have had a similar upbringing to other people your age. However, your parents and other influential people in your life will influence your outlook, so in some respects we are all very different and this is where it can get tricky.

You may have very different views to some of your friends and family, but that doesn't mean that yours are any more valid than another person, and whilst we do tend to gravitate to people who share our own values in life (see Build Your Tribe), there will be times when you will encounter people who have an opposing view to yours – and that's OK. In fact it's quite healthy to hear another person's reasoning of their views and opinions.

What isn't healthy though is to force your beliefs on to another person. They have every right to think the way they do, just as you do. You wouldn't like it if another person told you that you were wrong in your thinking, just as it's not wise to try to educate someone else to believe in what you believe in.

So long as you're not hurting anyone else, you do you and let others do them. It's fine to have a healthy debate about our differences, so long as you don't feel the need to convert someone else to your way of thinking and think that their beliefs are not worthy. It's all about acceptance of other people. And the same applies the other way round. If someone vehemently disagrees with your beliefs and refuses to listen to your arguments, allow them to do their own thing, while you continue to live your happy ever after.

Build Your Tribe

Psychologists say that we are a combination of the five people we spend most of our time with, so it's important to find the right tribe for you, because otherwise you could end up being influenced by the people around you, and if they are not positive and empowering, you will eventually become just like them.

This is why it's so important to surround yourself with people who have your back and your best interests at heart. For many of us, we still have people in our lives who we met when we were a lot younger. These may be school/college friends, people who have been our neighbours for the past 15 years or people we work with, and we often establish friendships with them because we share something in common with them.

The thing with this sort of tribe is that aside from a single thing that connects us, such as we went to the same school, you need to ask yourself, would they be willing to help you bury a body? Not that I endorse bumping someone off, but could you count on these people in your tribe if your life depended on it? Probably not, which is why you need to rethink who you want in your tribe who is more than someone you once shared office space with.

I discovered a few years ago that my tribe consisted of a few people I went to school with, a neighbour who I'd lived next door to for 10 years and a few women I'd met in the playground at my daughter's school. Despite knowing these people for half of my life, there wasn't one I felt that I could go to if I was having an emergency. We were all very polite and friendly to each other, but there was no one who I felt I could share a secret with, let along rely on helping me to bury a body should the occasion arise.

This is when I had a tribe revue (see Defriending) and decided to slowly defriend most of them and rediscover who I wanted in my tribe.

I decided I only wanted people who could inspire me to be a better person, not someone who bemoaned everything bad about the world. I wanted a tribe who would be there on the ground, cheering me on to skydive out of a plane, not someone who would tell me that my parachute would probably fail to deploy. I wanted people who were positive and full of energy, not people who would point out negative statistics at every opportunity.

And, you know what? I think I've got my tribe just right now. I have a very small group of people who I know will be there if I ring them up at 3 o'clock in the morning because I can't sleep because Dr Google has told me that a headache could be a brain aneurism. I have a tribe of people who would happily act as my alibi if I ever needed one and who push me to be the best I can be.

Think about who you want in your tribe, and you will soon attract the right people for you. People who will empower and genuinely want the best for you and for who you can do the same.

What's the Best That Can Happen?

When we're faced with life's challenges we're often reminded, what's the worst that can happen? The problem I have with this advice is that it can often lead to overthinking a situation and leave us expecting the worst possible outcome, making us feel anxious.

We will mull over a problem, thinking about the worst thing that will be the outcome. It's a kind of worry that is really not necessary and doesn't have any benefits to it. We think about that interview coming up, and think, well, what's the worst that can happen? I could make a complete fool out of myself, or they will see I've embellished the truth a little on my CV. The minute we start thinking about what the worse outcome will be is the minute the worries set in, and we begin to doubt ourselves and our abilities.

There's a philosophy within the Law of Attraction that says that our thoughts become things. The theory is that whatever we are thinking about, we are bringing it into our lives. Instead of thinking what's the worst that can happen, if we think, what's the best that can happen, our brains shift into assuming the very best and we attract the best possible outcomes.

99% of what we worry about doesn't actually happen, so wondering and worrying about the worst thing that can happen in a situation really is a waste of time, because all we're doing is making ourselves miserable and anxious by worrying about it. Added to this, the more power we give to the negatives of a problem, the more we will attract those negatives into our lives.

When we think what's the best that can happen, it shifts our energy from a negative outcome to a positive one. It also shows that we have faith in our own beliefs and take account for ourselves. When you think that 99% of the time the thing you were worrying about wasn't half as bad as you thought it was going to be, it makes sense to turn it on its head and wonder what the best that could happen could be.

You can adopt this attitude to any area of your life too. Worried that someone you like hasn't responded to your text? Instead of thinking what's the worst that could happen – he/she has ghosted you and you'll never hear from them again, you could think, what's the best that could happen? They've lost their phone or have a problem they have to fix and will get back to you soon; or even if they have chosen to ghost you, it could actually be for the best because they could have turned out to be a complete lunatic under that guise of beauty and you will have had a lucky escape.

Worrying about that interview coming up or expecting to fail that exam? What if you consider the best possible outcome? You actually turn out to be the ideal candidate or you nail that exam with plenty of time to spare. This not only makes you feel that you can accomplish anything you want in life, it's like a sign from the universe saying, I told you it would all work out, and you haven't spent time agonising over what the worst outcome might be.

If you are to live your happy ever after, it's much better for your health to consider what's the best that can happen.

Boundaries Can Become Cages

We're all familiar with the idea that we should set boundaries to protect ourselves from being hurt by others, but have you ever thought that those boundaries you set yourself could actually prevent you from having your best life?

We don't start life with boundaries set; rather we tend to set boundaries when something has happened that has caused us pain and we vow never to allow ourselves to be put in that position again, so we build up boundaries so that we won't ever become so vulnerable again.

The problem with doing this is that we can lose out on opportunities that might come our way simply because we remember the last time something like this happened. For example, you may have spent years wearing your heart on your sleeve, only to have it broken over and over again. Your natural instinct will be to never allow another person access to your true feelings, or at the very least, be very wary of letting another person fully into your life.

Whilst this is a natural response, it's also one that can keep us stuck in a rut. The boundaries that we put up to protect ourselves can become cages, preventing us from trying new things. Take for example, you decide to join a local book group. You love reading and think it would do you good to get out and meet other booky enthusiasts. When you get there, however, you feel like an outsider. All the other members already know each other, and they all seem far more intelligent than you. When they ask you who your favourite author is and you say JK Rowling, you can feel the sniggers behind the polite smiles, and you feel so uncomfortable that you vow never to return.

The next time you see a book club advertised, your automatic reaction would be to avoid it because of your previous experience of attending one. You don't want to experience feeling like an outsider or the joke of the group, like you did the last time you attended a book club, so you decide not to join another one.

Your boundary of not putting yourself in that position again has in fact caged you because now you won't get to experience what could be a wonderful evening with wonderful people who share the same interest as you do.

The same applies to when we get hurt by someone we love. Our 'once bitten' attitude could affect going out there and meeting someone else who will love us and meet all our expectations.

In order to live your happy ever after, put any bad experiences down to just that – a bad experience. You could be missing out on some wonderful opportunities in the future.

Life is Just a Series of Chapters

Much like a novel, your life is a series of chapters. Some of them are going to be rubbish, and others, well you just don't want them to end.

It's important to remember that every chapter in your life will have an expiry date. Things cannot possibly stay the same, just as you can't permanently feel sad or happy all the time. When life seems as though it's just one obstacle after another, it can be hard to see any light at the end of the tunnel or see that things will get better, but they always do.

When you think of your life as a fictitious story or a movie, you feel that you can call the shots as to what the next chapter/ scene is going to look like. It may sound like a cliché, but you really are the author or the director of what happens next in your life.

Every person in your life is a sub-character to your plot and this means that you can give them as much or as little attention as you wish. There will have been sub-characters you were very close to in some chapters in your life that have moved on and are no longer relevant to the plot. This might be because they've outstayed their welcome, or you've just outgrown them, but either way, they are no longer part of your story, so you can start a new chapter without them.

As we progress through life, we go through many chapters, and we need to do this in order to grow and experience new things. We can't remain a child under the care of our parents for ever because they have their own chapters to get through, and of course over time they age, so we have to leave them behind eventually and begin the next chapter, going to college or university and seeing how that chapter works out.

For many women one of the most challenging chapters of their lives is when their children leave home, and after many years of caring for them, they are suddenly faced with the prospect that they are no longer needed to be on call for their children and now have to start a whole new chapter. Many women who might have given up work in order to care for their children might feel at a loss as to what to do next, but as you're the author and storyteller, that's entirely up to you now.

My youngest daughter has recently flown my nest and just started university, and even though I've always worked, I can't tell you just how much this chapter in her life has affected this chapter in my life. I've had to learn that we both need to start a new chapter in order for her to grow and experience new things, but boy has it killed me at times!

There are no rules as to what can and can't be in the next chapter. Just as if you were writing about the journey of a character in a book, you can be that character and if you want your character to change career, travel the world, build a school for orphaned children, or become a best-selling author, you are in charge of your chapters, so why not include that in your life story?

An interesting observation is that when you decide to be in charge of the chapters of your life, other people who are used to the way you are, complain that you've changed. Spoiler alert! We're meant to change. Just as my daughters are not meant to continue living and relying on me, we're not meant to stay in one place or stay with the same people forevermore.

Every good book has many changes in it to keep the reader engaged and interested, and if you are going to live a happy and fulfilling life, this means you are going to have to make the changes that you want to see in your life. Some of them are going to be mistakes you wish you hadn't written and yet others are going to be the best chapters in your book of life or your screenplay. But either way, you are not a tree and you're not meant to stand still. You're meant to move and change as you go through life.

Wouldn't it be good to look back and see that each and every chapter made us grow and made us get the very best out of our life, rather than have a boring ending? And the best bit is, YOU get to write the story!

Eat Whatever The Hell You Want!

This may come as a shock to some, but you're a grown woman and you *are* allowed to eat what the hell you want, whenever you want!

A friend of mine called me the other day and whispered into the phone: "You'll never guess where I am? I'm in McDonald's and I'm having a Big Mac, fries and an apple pie."

I asked her why she was whispering, and she said, "I don't know, but don't tell Graham!"

Graham is my friend's husband and is a man completely obsessed with only eating a plant-based, healthy diet and woe-be-tide anyone who lets a morsel of fast-food pass their lips. Graham will feel obliged to tell you not only how many calories are in your food, but he will also point out how fatty your liver will become if you so much as look at a French fry and then demonstrate how many burpees he can do in under a minute. I suspect Graham is a closet binger.

Another friend feels she is a failure if she doesn't cook a daily meal from scratch for her family, and someone I used to regularly go out to lunch with, would tut-tut if I ordered a Coke to drink and proceed to send links to my phone about how cola rots your insides and turns your brain into jelly – whilst eating lunch. I mean WTAF?

First and foremost, if you are one of these people, please stop. What do you think gives you the right to belittle another person about what they choose to eat or drink? Secondly, we're all grown-ups here and are more than capable to educate ourselves as to what is considered to be a healthy diet or not.

Thirdly, I would never in a million years ever think about commenting on what someone else is eating or drinking. What right do I have to question how many calories someone else consumes? Frankly, I couldn't care less, Graham!

You're not a child and I'm sure you're equally aware that if you eat unhealthy food for every meal, you'll put on weight and possibly develop diabetes. You are a grown woman and therefore responsible and accountable to your eating choices. If that means you want to eat cereal for every meal, that's entirely up to you. It's no one else's business if you don't have your five fruit and veg every day or get your recommended 56 grams of daily protein.

Our bodies are amazing tools and will fortunately let us know when we are missing any important nutrients. Obviously I'm not promoting that you live off hamburgers and apple pies for ever, but if that's your choice, then who am I to tell you otherwise? Just as if you prefer to eat salad with every meal – entirely up to you. I don't care.

A colleague of mine used to shake her head whenever I drank sparkling bottled water, as if it was the devil's choice of beverage. "You drink a lot of that stuff, don't you?" she said one day. "Surely plain water is better for you?" Now, this is the woman who would drink at least 15 coffees a day and did I ever comment on the amount of caffeine she was consuming? No, because I really couldn't give a sh*t what she drank or ate.

The same woman was aghast that I don't cook meals, and at one point I thought she was going to have a heart attack when she discovered that Just Eat is on speed dial on my phone, and I ordered a takeout roast dinner for Christmas lunch. I don't enjoy cooking, my family are grown up and can cook for themselves now and... oh yes, I'm a grown woman who can eat or not eat whatever the hell I want.

When you feel like a chocolate bar, don't feel like you're being naughty, just have one and enjoy it. Don't feel that you have to tell everyone that you only eat seaweed for breakfast, dinner, and tea – no one cares, or if they do, then it just goes to show how very shallow they are.

You, as a grown woman, are entitled to eat whatever the hell you want, free from judgement from the Grahams of this world. In order to live your happy ever after, if anyone criticises or judges your eating habits, tell them to do one and enjoy that box of Ferrero Rocher for dinner!

(Don't) Act Your Age

Oh, so many rules we feel we must adhere to as women and here's another one – being told to act our age or be 'age appropriate', whether that be in the way we dress or how we talk or how we behave in public.

Why?

Why, just because we're grown-up women, should we act our age? Who gets to decide this? Who decides that once you reach a certain age you shouldn't be seen roller skating in the park or dancing in a nightclub?

And this rule about acting your age doesn't seem to apply to the opposite sex, does it? Have you ever watched the crowd at a football or a cricket match? Grown men dressed up in chicken costumes shouting and dancing in the stands or taking their tops off and wobbling their bellies in each other's faces. So don't give me this 'act your age' nonsense!

Our age is just the number of years we've been alive on this planet. It means diddly-squat to how you should behave, dress, talk or act. If you want to cover your body in tattoos, get your nose pierced, colour your hair fifty shades of pink, take up skateboarding or go and play on the swings in the park, do it. You don't need anyone's permission and you certainly don't need to be a certain age.

The TV presenter Carol Vorderman, who is in her sixties, constantly gets abuse for dressing the way she does – and surprisingly it's very often other women who are the abusers. So much for sisterhood eh? Carol works hard at maintaining a healthy body and often posts pictures of herself in skin-tight clothes. She always looks beautiful, but every time she posts a photo, she will get told to act her age and dress more appropriately.

Why the hell should she just because someone feels threatened by how beautiful she is? Even if she wasn't stunning, what gives someone else the right to tell another woman to act her age?

And what is acting your age anyway? It's conforming to how other people assume a person of a certain age should behave and this is very subjective. The previous generations' ideas on how a person's age should affect how they act/dress/behave would have been that any woman over the age of fifty should wear an apron and have a home perm at all times.

It is the women like Carol Vorderman, Iris Apfel, Cyndi Lauper, Debbie Harry, and Vivienne Westwood, who refuse to believe in acting their age who are an inspiration to women across the world.

Regardless of your age, you have permission to act however you want. Don't let society tell you otherwise, and to those who tell you that you should act your age, tell them to get stuffed. You will be the one still having fun in your eighties and beyond!

Be Unpredictable

I was listening to a podcast the other day, and it was about why unpredictable women are more interesting to men and why by being unpredictable keeps people on their toes. Now, whilst I'm not here to promote dating tips, I believe this is good advice for every area in your life.

When we're predictable we give the impression that we will always be seen as the reliable one that others can count on in times of need. When we are predictable, other people know that they can behave badly and get away with it because we always forgive them, or we will be the one who remembers your partner's mother's birthday and will get a card and present – and sign it from them. We will always be the one who will pick out the best restaurant to eat at or arrange the holiday accommodation, including transfers.

Jane, a friend of mine, recently said, "I am sick and tired of being the one who always organises family events. I hate that I'm expected to find a place to eat, book a reservation and everyone else just rocks up and enjoys themselves! For once it would be nice to not be the one who predictably organises every family get-together!"

I asked her why she just doesn't do it, and she said that everyone expects her to.

So what do you think would happen if Jane decided that she wasn't going to organise the next family event? Jane said that nothing would get booked and that the family wouldn't meet up. So the only reason why Jane's family all get together is because they all know that she will organise everything for them.

When Jane stopped doing this, nobody died, there was no massive family fallout. They were a little bemused as to why Jane hadn't organised anything for Christmas that year, but they all managed to sort something out, and realised just how difficult it was to get everyone together on a certain date, giving Jane the respect she rightly deserved.

When you stop being predictable, people sit up and take notice of you. Just as we discussed in the previous chapter on not having to feel you have to justify your actions, when you stop being predictable, you don't have to explain why. Just stop doing what you've always been doing. Stop being the first person to text or call. Stop being the first one to make arrangements. Stop being the first one to apologise, and stop being the first one to make amends.

You will be amazed at how when you are unpredictable, other people begin to respect you more. Obviously you don't want to become one of those people who you never know if they're going to be in a good mood or a bad mood whenever they see you – that's just taking it to the extremes and people will avoid you. But you don't have to always be the one who does everything for everyone else. You don't have to make a roast dinner every Sunday or have everyone over for Christmas if you don't want to. You don't have to be the first one to say sorry after an argument. You can take yourself off to the cinema on your own one afternoon if you feel like it.

Whatever has become the norm for you, why not shake it up a little and be a little bit unpredictable?

Nah, I'm Not Having It!

This is a saying I've recently adopted (I might just get a T-shirt printed), and in order to live your happy ever after, I urge you to do the same.

Throughout our lives we have to deal with some people who are rude, argumentative, or just downright annoying, and do you know what? You don't have to put up with it. You can say, "Nah, I'm not having it!"

I've been using this phrase a lot and you'll be surprised at how empowering it is to declare this out loud. Unfortunately, in this day and age, many people act and behave in ways where they think they can do and say whatever they want with no accountability or recompense. Whether this is something they say on social media, or something they say or do in person that offends or annoys you, you don't have to put up with it. If you feel that something is unjust, tell yourself you're not having it and that you deserve to be treated better than this.

You can apply this phrase to anything in your life:

You take a friend out to lunch, and they do nothing but moan about the meal, are rude to the staff and everything that comes out of their mouth is negative. This actually happened to me recently, and by the end of the meal I felt so angry and miserable that I thought, nah, I'm not having it, and I paid the bill and walked out. I don't want to spend an hour in someone else's company if the experience is going to make me feel miserable and angry.

Or perhaps your insurance company has automatically renewed a policy you cancelled, and they won't refund it? Nah, I'm not having it! Get on the phone and demand to speak to the MD of the company. It may well be a computer error, but someone somewhere is accountable – computers don't yet work without someone putting the necessary coding and information in them.

If your partner has a habit of talking over you in a conversation and ignores your voice, say, nah, I'm not having it! Calmly ask why they feel their voice is more important than yours. You don't have to raise your voice – in fact, the calmer you can remain, the better.

If someone tries to belittle you in front of other people, think to yourself, nah, I'm not having this and call them out on it. Don't just laugh it off again. Ask them why they feel the need to make you look small and stupid in front of everyone, and do this in front of the very people they have tried making you look small to.

When someone replies to one of your social media posts and tries to make you look inferior, call them out. Say, nah, I'm not having it, and politely ask them why they did it. Everyone is entitled to their opinion, but at the same time, everyone is entitled to be respected, and unfortunately very few people are held accountable for their actions.

When you decide that you're not having it, you are setting boundaries to other people as to how much bullsh*t you will take from them. You are not a doormat, and you have every right to call people out if you feel they are rude to you.

It takes a bit of practice to make this a way of life. Many women feel incapable of voicing what they really want to say for fear of being thought of as a bad person, which again comes from our childhood conditioning – good girls shouldn't make a fuss, good girls shouldn't be assertive; it's not attractive, blah, blah, blah. So we should all be doormats and let people walk all over us and say and do whatever they feel like, should we? Nah, I'm not having that!

When you question why someone feels that they have the right to dismiss you, be rude or angry with you, or feel that they can get away with things they wouldn't with other people, a strange thing happens. The offender will often make up an excuse, or say you're being too sensitive, and you can't take a joke. This is the time to ask them again why they felt their actions were necessary. Suddenly they don't feel so confident.

Like my lunch guest, they might just not contact you again, and that's OK. You don't need people like that in your life. In the case of anything to do with a company overcharging you, you will receive an apology and the problem will be rectified.

You are not being aggressive when you say, nah, I'm not having it. You are being assertive, and you are putting your foot down, and you have absolutely every right to do that. In fact it's necessary for you to live happily ever after.

You Are Enough

If I had one wish it would be for every woman to accept that she is enough just as she is. In a world where we are bombarded by pictures of perfection on a daily basis, whether that is to have the perfect body, the perfect hair, the perfect style, it's easy to feel inferior and less than.

I'm here to tell you that YOU ARE ENOUGH! You are perfect just the way you are, and I know that's hard to believe, but did you know the fact that you were born is a miracle in itself. It's a billions to one chance that you were even born. When you think of the chances of your parents meeting and liking each other enough to have a relationship and become parents, it's amazing that you are even here at all!

As women we are fed so much false information that little by little it chips away at our self-esteem and confidence; it's no wonder we never feel as though we're enough. We are constantly judged on what we 'should' be doing – we 'should' be this or that at such and such an age. We 'should' get married, we 'should' have babies, we 'should' be able to juggle working full time, bringing up a family, making cakes worthy of a *Great British Bake Off* winner and look like we've just stepped out of the cover of *Vogue* magazine all at the same time – oh and have an immaculate home to boot!

Is it any wonder why the majority of women feel they are not enough? You are more than enough. You are amazing, and whilst I'm a firm believer in going for your goals, whatever they might be, I'm also a firm believer in telling yourself that right now, you are enough, just as you are.

The fantastic motivational guru Mel Robbins emphasises this in her book, *The High 5 Habit*. Mel is committed to helping women realise that they are enough, and I urge anyone feeling that they're not to look her up and buy her books because she will make you realise just how important you are right now, whatever stage you are at in life.

If you have children it's important to remember that they will pick up on your little 'I hate me' traits that you say to yourself on a daily basis. Those comments such as, "God, I look awful this morning" and "I'm rubbish at technology", all these micro statements are picked up by your children and others around you.

Just as we know from our own childhoods, we subconsciously adopt the negative beliefs our parents say about themselves, and they eventually become our negative beliefs. If you have a mother who was constantly putting herself down and saying she was not good enough, you will automatically take on those beliefs as your own.

Now is the time to stop and remind yourself that you are enough just as you are, because you are. It doesn't matter if you're not the prettiest, the smartest, the world's best cake maker or you can't work out the new menu on the TV. You are still enough!

In order to live your happy ever after, stop comparing yourself to other people, because guess what? They're doing exactly the same with you. Accept that you are enough right here, right now, and if you want to work on a particular area in your life, then by all means do it, but because you want to be the new improved version of you, not because you feel dissatisfied with who you are right now.

Perfect Day

If you remember in a previous chapter, we spoke about acting as if you are the person you eventually want to become. Well, this chapter is an extension of that and one that always makes me feel happy because it's about thinking about what your perfect day would be, writing it down and reading it over and over again to yourself. You can't help but feel happy vibes when you do this, and if you don't then you need to go back and rewrite it until you do.

When we think about our goals we tend to think about one particular goal at a time. For example, you might want to get the latest BMW or move to the countryside, or get a promotion at work, or study to become a forensic scientist, or get married, have children, live on your own after your children have moved out. Whatever your goals are, we all think about them as a separate entity and don't tend to think how they will be incorporated into our daily lives.

When you tie your goals into your perfect day, you make them more attainable because you can actually imagine how all these different goals will have an impact on your daily living.

So, let's say you want to live in a little cottage, start your own candle-making business and be so successful that you can afford your own premises, hire staff, and afford to buy that cute VW Campervan you have your eye on to go travelling in. And you want a really lovely partner to share it all with.

Get a nice new notebook and start writing what your perfect day would look like. In the above example, it might read something like this…

It's 9am in the morning and I wake up to the sound of the birds chattering away outside. I wake feeling relaxed from a good night's sleep in my beautiful two-bed cottage in the middle of the countryside.

I wash and dress and feel excited for the day ahead because I have a new batch of essential oils arriving today for my business, Candy Candles. Once dressed (I always look stunning), I eat my breakfast of croissant and orange juice in my patio garden and feel the early morning sun on my skin, invigorating me for the day.

I take the short stroll to my shop. It's already busy with customers which my wonderful staff deal with and I can just about keep up with the orders and sales coming in every day; soon I will have to take on more staff. I spend the next few hours talking to customers and creating new scented candles until at lunchtime when I leave the shop in my staff's capable hands and meet a friend Paris for lunch at our local pub.

In the afternoon I make even more sales and create more candles in my workshop adjacent to the shop. After closing up, I meet my lovely new partner (insert details of what he/she is like) for dinner, and I am wined and dined, and we have the best time. I always feel so loved. I leave the restaurant early because I have to get up in the morning to catch the ferry with Mildred, my beautiful campervan, for three glorious weeks driving around Europe on my own…

Can you see the difference between just writing down what things you want and actually detailing them so that they become your lifestyle? When we just write that we want a new car, we're not being specific about how we will use that new car, or how it will play in our lives in the future. It's just a sentence of what you want. Oftentimes we say we want a particular thing, say the latest iPhone, but when we get it we feel dissatisfied because, well, it's just another phone.

When we imagine how we will use that new phone, how we'll be able to download our emails, social media apps and basically everything we would need so that we won't have to be tied to our desks all day long and can run our business with it, that new phone becomes something that we get excited about because we're implementing it into our daily life.

This is such a fun exercise to do, and when you read your Perfect Day back to yourself over and over again, you are more likely to believe that you can attain anything that you want and live that perfect day, every day. It's very important that you write your perfect day as if you were living it right now – remember: your brain can't distinguish between whether what you imagine is real or not!

Give it a go. Trust me, you can't help but smile when you read back what you've written. If you think this is all a bit woo-woo then by all means go back to living the life you already live, but what if it does work? What if you could live your perfect day every day?

Thank You!

And while we're on about creating our perfect life, did you know that the quickest way to help you get your ideal life is to be grateful for what you already have right now?

Best-selling author Rhonda Byrne's books, *The Secret*, *The Power*, and *The Magic* all detail how practising gratitude on a daily basis will propel us forwards to having everything we want in the future. If we're not thankful for what we already have, right here and now, we send out an ungrateful energy, and we will miss out on so many future opportunities that will move us forwards to the life we want to lead.

I don't have room to go into great detail about the science behind the gratitude theory, but when you are thankful and you combine that with the belief that you will get the life you want, these are very powerful thoughts that enter your subconscious.

While you might think it silly that by just saying thanks and believing that you can get anything you want you will manifest it, think about electricity for example. You can't see it and yet you believe that when you flick a light switch the light will come on.

It's suggested that you should make being thankful a daily habit and write down at least 10 things that you are thankful for every single day. Even if you're not having the best of times there is always something to be thankful for. For starters you woke up this morning still breathing. You have a roof over your head. You have electricity, gas, and water. You have food in the cupboards. You have a computer or a phone. You have clothes to wear etc. You have this book to read. Hell, given that our planet only survives because it is in the right place at the right time in the universe, we should be eternally grateful that we are here at all! Once you start you can list literally hundreds of things to be thankful for every day.

Added to this, it's impossible to feel unhappy when you start listing what you already have to be thankful for. There have been times when I simply haven't bothered to do my daily gratitude list because I'm having a massive pity party and I've noticed that when I don't do my list, I feel miserable, angry, and unhappy and things always go wrong for me.

When I start being grateful again – and sometimes I have to force myself to keep it up – my world becomes a much better place. I get more opportunities and seem to be able to knock down any obstacles in my way. Things I want to happen, just happen.

In addition to doing your daily thankful list, you could also list things that you don't yet have but you plan to have at some point. So if you want a new car, you will write how thankful you are for your new Porsche (or car of preference).

Try it and you will soon see your life moving forwards, and you deserve it in order to live your happy ever after!

Sorry, not Sorry…

I come from a long line of chronic apologisers on my mum's side. We apologise if we call someone and they're in the middle of something. We apologise if someone's sick or if they're having a bad day. Damn, we even apologise to the door we walk into!

It's only when a friend got cross with me for apologising because her dog had died – "You didn't kill it, did you!" was her actual response – did I realise just how annoying it is to other people to be the one saying sorry all the time. I say sorry even when I have nothing to be sorry for. Sometimes, I apologise for even being alive, and yes, it is very, very annoying, not only to me, but to the people around me.

If you think you're also an avid apologiser, then I want you to take the page from this book and stop doing it, even if something is your fault – STOP SAYING I'M SORRY!

Apologising for something that you have no reason to apologise for just rubs people up the wrong way. A friend's having a bad day – you apologise to them. Your son's car broke down – you apologise to them. You call in sick at work – and you apologise for being sick. You missed someone's call – you apologise that you missed it, even though you were on the loo at the time, and it was an inconvenient time for you to take the call. Yes, this is me too.

But think about it for a moment. You didn't create your friend's bad day, so why are you apologising? You didn't break your son's car and you can't help but be sick enough to take a day off work. You have a life and can't be tied to your phone just on the off chance someone will call you – we all need to poop at some point!

Why do we do this?

According to psychologists, people who apologise for things that they have no control over, for example, when it's raining and your colleague gets wet or you apologise to your friends for your partner's grumpy behaviour, it's because some of us are wired to overcompensate and make other people feel better about themselves. Women in particular are raised to be considerate of others' feelings and often apologise even when something is nothing to do with us because we feel it shows that we empathise with the other person in some way. It's also a sign that we don't believe in our own self-worth.

We will often apologise for wasting or interrupting someone else's time – "I'm sorry to bother you, but could you tell me where the accounts department it?"

I've slowly learned to train myself to stop apologising for existing, for other people's behaviours, bad moods, that I missed their call and to the lamppost I just walked in to. Because it's actually not my fault.

Obviously it's just good manners to apologise if you've hurt someone in some way, but when it gets to the point where you are apologising for even breathing the same air as someone, all it is doing is showing the other person that they are above you.

So, here's a few tips I've learned to do instead of saying I'm sorry...

- If you're late to meet someone.
  Instead of apologising, say, "Thanks for waiting for me."
- If your friend's dog has died.
  Instead of apologising, say, "I'm here if you need to cry."
- If you miss someone's call.
  Instead of apologising, just call them back.
- If your partner behaves badly or is rude when you're out.
  Instead of apologising, say, "I think *you* should apologise for the way you behaved."
- If you need information from someone.
  Instead of apologising for bothering them, say, "Can you help me?"

I'm not saying it's easy when you've been a chronic apologiser all your life, but you really have no reason to be sorry for anything that is out of your control, or when you haven't played a part in upsetting someone.

Do other people apologise to you for breathing too loud or calling you when it's inconvenient? No, they don't. So why should you always feel as though you should apologise? In order to live your happy ever after, stop saying I'm sorry to everyone. You are just as worthy as anyone else in this world, and you really do not have to apologise for something you have no control over.

Never Chase Someone...

Just as we talked about why when you treat someone like a celebrity, you will always be their fan, you should never feel the need to chase another person.

Whether it's a friend, a romantic relationship, or a family member, you do not need to be the one chasing them, because when you do, you are giving them power over how they treat you in the future.

Let's say you've been asked out to dinner by someone you really like. The date has been great, and you think, finally, I've met my soulmate! You agree to see each other again soon but don't make any arrangements that night.

As tempting as it is, this is not the time to go home, change into your PJs and start bombarding them with messages, or calling them to see when you are going to see them again. Once again, this puts you in the position of being their fan. The minute you begin to chase someone the dynamics of the relationship will change. You will no longer be seen as equal. You will have become the chaser.

Now, I know you could argue that someone has to make the first move – they do, but it doesn't have to be YOU.

If someone wants to be with you, they will move heaven and earth to be with you. You do not have to persuade another person that you are worthy of being in their lives and you certainly do not have to chase after them. Relationship experts call this being 'the convincer'.

When you chase someone – always the first to text, always the one to suggest meeting up, always the one to initiate intimacy – you are trying to convince the other person that you are worthy of their love and affection. This is a massive turn off to other people.

Think of it like this, how do you feel if a salesperson

constantly bombards you with calls, messages, or emails about how you can save money by switching your home insurance? It just makes you feel as though they won't leave you alone. It certainly doesn't make you want to buy their insurance plan.

It's exactly the same principle. It doesn't matter how compatible you think you and another person are, or how you feel they're your soulmate and you're destined to be together for eternity; when you voice how you feel, you are coming from a place of neediness and trying to convince the other person.

People don't like being convinced; they like to be able to make up their own minds about something, and the funny thing is, the minute you just allow something to be or not be, the other person will come to you of their own accord – or they might not. It doesn't matter either way because when you don't feel the need to chase someone and you come from a place of, meh, can take it or leave it, you live your happy ever after which is not reliant on anybody else's interest in you.

If It Only Takes Five Minutes, Do It…

I was once asked to write a piece for a magazine about time management and how women often get frustrated that they don't have enough time in their lives to do everything. One lady I interviewed told me, "If something takes five minutes or less, I'll do it there and then." And I've lived by this advice ever since.

Like most women I don't have the luxury of a housekeeper, cleaner, cook, washer-upper, lunch box packer, chauffeur, problem solver, bill payer; and even if you do have a partner to share the load of simply living, rarely do the chores and general day-to-day things get shared equally unfortunately.

When you use the 'Five Minute' rule, it actually makes your life a lot easier than getting to the end of the week and realising that you have a list as long as your arm of things you have to do which will eat into your weekend.

Day-to-day things to do mount up – the curtain pole has fallen down, the bathroom bin is overflowing, the toilet roll hasn't been put into the holder, your desk is a mountain of paperwork, you need to call the plumber, you haven't RSVP'd that invite to your friend's birthday do… see it all adds up!

All the above can be done in less than five minutes. Start by jotting down all the things that need doing in your life, then break them down into jobs that will take no longer than five minutes. Anything that will take longer, such as filing your yearly accounts, or getting round to putting the guest-bed together, can be put onto another list.

You'll be amazed at how much you can actually get done in five minutes. For example, you can load the dishwasher, wipe the sides down and put the condiments away all within five minutes every evening, resulting in you having a lovely clean kitchen to wake up to for breakfast in the morning. When you're running a bath in the evening, you can spend the five minutes you're waiting for the tub to fill by putting the towels away or emptying the bathroom bin. If you need to make a dental appointment, get hold of a gas engineer, and book an appointment with your hairdresser, you can dedicate the five minutes you're waiting for the kettle to boil to do all three. When I'm swishing my mouth with mouthwash, I clean the sink at the same time – boom, two jobs done in one go!

I've found that when I apply the 'Five Minute' rule, most of the things I have on my to-do list can be done, freeing up my time for stuff I enjoy doing, rather than spending my free time catching up on chores.

Journaling…

In the good ole days it was called writing a diary, but today we call it journaling and it really is a godsend to anyone who wants to find their happy ever after, and I'll tell you for why…

When you write down what's going on in your life it helps you to process your thoughts and feelings without having to voice them to someone else. When you get into the habit of journaling, it feels as though you are no longer alone in your thoughts. You feel as though you have someone to talk to without actually having to talk to someone.

Studies have shown that when we write our thoughts down on paper, our brain can process them better, because by doing something practical, we're releasing the thoughts. This prevents us from overthinking because our brains associate the action of writing with completion. A bit like when you write a shopping list – if we try to remember everything we need to buy from the store in our head we invariably forget something. When we write a list, we have a physical reference to refer to, and our brain doesn't need to work to remember it over and over again.

Added to this, oftentimes what goes around inside our heads, we think we couldn't possibly say out loud to anyone – like those times when you imagine being Michael Douglas' character in *Falling Down* after you've heard 'unrecognisable item in the bagging area, please remove it' one too many times.

Evidence suggests that journaling is a very good idea if you want to live your happy ever after, and the best thing is it doesn't cost very much at all – basically a notebook and a pen/pencil. I always find it pays to find a nice quality notebook because it's going to be something you write in and refer to again and again, so treat yourself to something nice.

Despite what many will tell you, there really are no rules to journaling. You can add stickers, doodle, draw in it, hell, cover it in gold glitter if that makes you feel good! The main thing is that you use it to write down your thoughts and feelings – and you don't need to hold back. Every emotion is a valid emotion. If you're feeling angry because the recycling truck didn't empty your bin because there was a rogue non-recyclable two-minute rice container in it, write it down. If you had a moment of happiness because you discovered there was one of your favourite biscuits left in the cookie jar, write it down.

You may be going through a tough time right now and that's perfectly normal but write down how you are feeling. Bottling it up is the worst thing you can do when you're feeling a multitude of emotions, and we all need somewhere to release them.

As I mentioned in the It Will Pass – Honestly! chapter, when you get into the habit of journaling, you will be able to look back at the sh*tty times and realise just how far you've come. You'll see that time when you lost the job you loved so much, or you felt destroyed when the one you loved more than anything in the world walked out of your life, or the time your child told you they hated you and wished you were dead; they all passed, and you recovered from those events. You will realise that you've survived some sh*t in the past and you will survive it again if you have to.

It's also nice to look back on the past years and see how what might have been bothering you doesn't now. Some people worry that if they write their real thoughts down, someone might read it and get upset. I say, it's curiosity that killed the cat, and if they can't respect your privacy, then that's a them problem.

There is an alternative if you are worried about someone accessing your real thoughts and that's to use a website called Future Me (www.futureme.org). This is a secure website where you can write a letter to your future self for free and it's delivered electronically to your email on the date you choose it to be delivered to you.

I use a combination of both a hard copy journal and the Future

Me one because I think it's nice to receive a letter detailing what my life was like five years ago and what was bothering me at the time. I know other women who devise their own code for their diaries with invented names of people who are in their lives right now, so that if that person decides to have a nose through they won't know they're being written about.

In order to live your happy ever after, grab a notebook and start journaling all your thoughts and feelings. You'll feel so much better when you do.

End Note...

Thank you for purchasing and reading this book, you beautiful lady you! It is my wish that every woman, regardless of who you are, finds and lives their happy ever after. When you realise that you are worthy of having a happy life and that you don't have to put up with bad behaviour from anyone or adhere to society's unspoken or spoken rules, you become a power to be reckoned with.

You are not obliged to be anything other than you and you don't need to listen to the naysayers who tell you that you should be doing this or should be doing that. This is YOUR life. You are unique and already perfect just as you are. You don't need to listen to the opinions or beliefs of anyone else if you don't want to.

You are a beautiful, powerful woman and you deserve to live happily ever after!

I still have so much to say on the subject of empowering women, so if you want to join other women who are determined to live their own happy ever after, please come and join us at And She Lived Happily Ever After HQ:

www.happyeverafter.org.uk

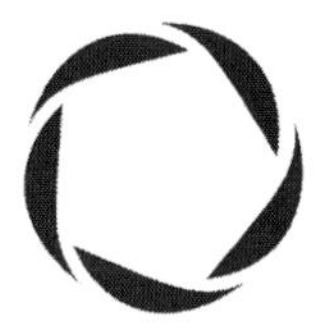

O-BOOKS

SPIRITUALITY

O is a symbol of the world, of oneness and unity; this eye represents knowledge and insight. We publish titles on general spirituality and living a spiritual life. We aim to inform and help you on your own journey in this life.
If you have enjoyed this book, why not tell other readers by posting a review on your preferred book site?

Recent bestsellers from O-Books are:

Heart of Tantric Sex

Diana Richardson

Revealing Eastern secrets of deep love and intimacy to Western couples.

Paperback: 978-1-90381-637-0 ebook: 978-1-84694-637-0

Crystal Prescriptions

The A-Z guide to over 1,200 symptoms and their healing crystals

Judy Hall

The first in the popular series of eight books, this handy little guide is packed as tight as a pill-bottle with crystal remedies for ailments.

Paperback: 978-1-90504-740-6 ebook: 978-1-84694-629-5

Take Me To Truth

Undoing the Ego

Nouk Sanchez, Tomas Vieira

The best-selling step-by-step book on shedding the Ego, using the teachings of *A Course In Miracles*.

Paperback: 978-1-84694-050-7 ebook: 978-1-84694-654-7

The 7 Myths about Love...Actually!

The Journey from your HEAD to the HEART of your SOUL

Mike George

Smashes all the myths about LOVE.

Paperback: 978-1-84694-288-4 ebook: 978-1-84694-682-0

The Holy Spirit's Interpretation of the New Testament
A Course in Understanding and Acceptance
Regina Dawn Akers
Following on from the strength of *A Course In Miracles*, NTI teaches us how to experience the love and oneness of God.
Paperback: 978-1-84694-085-9 ebook: 978-1-78099-083-5

The Message of A Course In Miracles
A translation of the Text in plain language
Elizabeth A. Cronkhite
A translation of *A Course in Miracles* into plain, everyday language for anyone seeking inner peace. The companion volume, *Practicing A Course In Miracles*, offers practical lessons and mentoring.
Paperback: 978-1-84694-319-5 ebook: 978-1-84694-642-4

Your Simple Path
Find Happiness in every step
Ian Tucker
A guide to helping us reconnect with what is really important in our lives.
Paperback: 978-1-78279-349-6 ebook: 978-1-78279-348-9

365 Days of Wisdom
Daily Messages To Inspire You Through The Year
Dadi Janki
Daily messages which cool the mind, warm the heart and guide you along your journey.
Paperback: 978-1-84694-863-3 ebook: 978-1-84694-864-0

Body of Wisdom

Women's Spiritual Power and How it Serves

Hilary Hart

Bringing together the dreams and experiences of women across the world with today's most visionary spiritual teachers.

Paperback: 978-1-78099-696-7 ebook: 978-1-78099-695-0

Dying to Be Free

From Enforced Secrecy to Near Death to True Transformation

Hannah Robinson

After an unexpected accident and near-death experience, Hannah Robinson found herself radically transforming her life, while a remarkable new insight altered her relationship with her father, a practising Catholic priest.

Paperback: 978-1-78535-254-6 ebook: 978-1-78535-255-3

The Ecology of the Soul

A Manual of Peace, Power and Personal Growth for Real People in the Real World

Aidan Walker

Balance your own inner Ecology of the Soul to regain your natural state of peace, power and wellbeing.

Paperback: 978-1-78279-850-7 ebook: 978-1-78279-849-1

Not I, Not other than I

The Life and Teachings of Russel Williams

Steve Taylor, Russel Williams

The miraculous life and inspiring teachings of one of the World's greatest living Sages.

Paperback: 978-1-78279-729-6 ebook: 978-1-78279-728-9

On the Other Side of Love

A woman's unconventional journey towards wisdom

Muriel Maufroy

When life has lost all meaning, what do you do?

Paperback: 978-1-78535-281-2 ebook: 978-1-78535-282-9

Practicing A Course In Miracles

A translation of the Workbook in plain language, with mentor's notes

Elizabeth A. Cronkhite

The practical second and third volumes of The Plain-Language *A Course In Miracles*.

Paperback: 978-1-84694-403-1 ebook: 978-1-78099-072-9

Quantum Bliss

The Quantum Mechanics of Happiness, Abundance, and Health

George S. Mentz

Quantum Bliss is the breakthrough summary of success and spirituality secrets that customers have been waiting for.

Paperback: 978-1-78535-203-4 ebook: 978-1-78535-204-1

The Upside Down Mountain

Mags MacKean

A must-read for anyone weary of chasing success and happiness – one woman's inspirational journey swapping the uphill slog for the downhill slope.

Paperback: 978-1-78535-171-6 ebook: 978-1-78535-172-3

Your Personal Tuning Fork

The Endocrine System

Deborah Bates

Discover your body's health secret, the endocrine system, and 'twang' your way to sustainable health!

Paperback: 978-1-84694-503-8 ebook: 978-1-78099-697-4